Kris Hallenga lives in Cornwall with her cat, Lady Marmalade. At twenty-three she was diagnosed with Stage 4, secondary, incurable cancer. She and her twin sister Maren founded the first breast cancer education charity, CoppaFeel!, which raises over £2 million per year, successfully campaigned to change the school curriculum, and has saved many lives. She has received a Pride of Britain Award, a Cosmopolitan Ultimate Campaigner Award, and been awarded an honorary doctorate from Nottingham Trent University. Kris stepped down as CEO six years ago and now pursues speaking engagements, writing and dipping in the cold sea while working for CoppaFeel! part time. Occasionally she even finds time to remember she has cancer.

Glittering a Turd

How surviving the unsurvivable taught me to live

KRIS HALLENGA

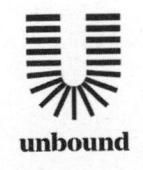

unbound

First published in 2021
This paperback edition first published in 2022

Unbound
Level 1, Devonshire House,
One Mayfair Place, London W1J 8AJ

www.unbound.com

Extracts from *When the Body Says No* by Gabor Maté published by
Vermilion. Copyright © Gabor Maté 2019. Reprinted by permission of The
Random House Group Limited.

While every effort has been made to trace the owners of copyright
material reproduced herein, the publisher would like to apologise for
any omissions and will be pleased to incorporate missing
acknowledgements in any further editions.

Text design by Ellipsis, Glasgow

A CIP record for this book is available from the British Library

ISBN 978-1-80018-177-9 (trade pbk)
ISBN 978-1-80018-231-8 (limited edition pbk)
ISBN 978-1-80018-048-2 (hbk)
ISBN 978-1-80018-049-9 (ebook)

Printed and bound by Clays Ltd, Elcograf S.p.A
1 3 5 7 9 8 6 4 2

For Herbie. For reassuring me that life can,
and will, go on.

'You can't polish a turd, but you can roll it in glitter'

Contents

Introduction

I did not expect to be diagnosed with breast cancer at twenty-three. I also did not expect to write a book about it during a global pandemic. But here we are. If there's something to learn from life (aside from its unpredictability) it's that turds come in varying shapes, sizes and guises. You might find this hard to believe after the shitshow that was 2020, but even the most unpolishable turds are glitterable – let's face it, that stuff gets everywhere. This is the story of someone who glittered hers (that's a plural – I got greedy) and decided it was worth sharing with the world in the hope it helps others find greater meaning too.

But I do have a tiny confession. I set off to write this book in a bid to help you, the reader, not really fully appreciating that it would help heal the one person I thought was already healed: me. I had every intention to write this purely for your sake (you're welcome), I wanted so badly to move people (like Oprah), but throughout the process I realised that I was doing the very thing that all this was supposed to have taught me I didn't need to do: namely, please others. My cancer diagnosis was a harsh lesson to stop expending all my energy on everything and everyone, and go inwards. This book forced me to do the same. This book has become a manual into my inner workings. This book helped me discover *me*. In aiming to show you all the meaning I'd discovered, all I found was the inner workings of yours truly.

However, on my journey to that epiphany I leave a trail of breadcrumbs (or glitter – you decide) that I think will help you too, because the truth is that we all have turds that need glittering, and sometimes it helps to follow someone's already trodden path. Are we done with the turd analogy now? OK, let's go . . .

The Turd

'Is there anyone here with you today?'

I thought that was a pretty odd question for the nurse to ask me as I waited for my breast clinic appointment on that Thursday morning in 2009. 'My mum's just coming,' I replied. 'She's parking the car.' As per usual, the car park was full and we Hallengas have a tendency to be on time to things – never early, not usually late, just on time – so it didn't give us the chance to hunt for a space before having to get to my appointment. That question was unsettling, but so too was our cat, Lucky, coming to sit on my lap before we left the house. This wasn't something he normally did, especially since he'd already been fed.

In her book *The Year of Magical Thinking*, Joan Didion writes 'confronted with sudden disaster we all focus on how unremarkable the circumstances were in which the unthinkable occurred'. Unremarkable maybe, but every aspect of that day is so vivid and so indelibly etched into my brain even now.

I was feeling a little the worse for wear. I'd spent the previous night in Birmingham with a friend getting unreasonably happy on midweek cocktails. The day before had been my dead father's birthday, and was also the anniversary of the day my sort-of-ex-boyfriend and I had got together a few years before. I was, in other words, drinking to forget. I wondered whether my sore head made me misjudge the weather and thus my outfit choice. For some reason I'd decided to wear a miniskirt, with tights and high boots and an oversized belt (a fashion faux pas I somehow forgot to leave in the 1990s), a T-shirt and a long cardigan that I'd bought at Urban Outfitters in the sale the day before. It was a windy, chilly day; it would be – it was February.

Without waiting for my mum to arrive, the nurse took me into the tiny, clinical consultation room. It was cold. I was cold. She sat me on the one and only chair. As I waited for the consultant to come in, I wondered where he would sit. Would he lean or sit on the bed? Or should I, as the patient, sit on the bed? I mean, was I even a patient? I wasn't sick. *This could get awkward*, I thought. Before I could make any seating changes, he walked in, with an unexpected entourage. There was a registrar and two nurses, making the already small room feel even more airless. We swiftly got through the pleasantries and on to the main event: biopsy results.

'I was concerned about the fact your grandma had breast cancer at a young age. I am sorry. It's not good news. You have breast cancer.'

WHAT.

JUST.

HAPPENED?

I was partly still stuck on the fact he was concerned about my grandma having breast cancer when she was thirty. When I'd first told him, he'd dismissed that detail pretty swiftly – it was apparently not a strong enough link; one family member isn't enough to increase risk. I couldn't bring this up with him now, though; in fact, I couldn't find any words at all. What could I possibly say? In my head I was saying *what?* and *shit* and *how?* again and again. I felt like my breath had been sucked out of me. I was sobbing; I felt nauseous; I felt faint; I wasn't really there. I was there physically, but somehow I was watching it all happen from outside of my body. I felt like a surveillance camera hanging from the corner of the room, capturing a life being shattered.

The next thing I knew, Mum was in the room. She could, of course, tell from my distraught face that I had just been told some pretty horrendous news. The doctor repeated what he'd told me. And Mum burst into tears. I remember her first words like I'm still there: 'It should be me, not you.'

In interviews it's always one of the first questions I get asked: 'How did it feel to be diagnosed?' But I don't really know – I can't describe it well enough. I mean, I could use a lot of expletives. One hundred and fifty women per day (that's about one woman every ten minutes) are told the same news I was told that day, and how I describe that moment would probably be no different from the way they would. It was simply *shit*. And more than that, it was baffling. I was baffled that this was the first time the word 'cancer' had come up, and my journey to this very moment made this all the more bewildering, too.

So let's rewind, shall we?

My relationship with my boobs was a pretty normal one. I could never understand the fuss girls made about having small ones or too-big ones. I guess I was lucky; I just had fairly normal-sized ones. My boobs and I were, in short, ticking along in life just fine. I never got a bra fitted; like many puberty topics that Mum never broached with us, the subject never came up, so it was more of a fend-for-yourself situation. So I made the (I thought) excellent decision to upgrade from my white vest to buying my first underwired bra from Next myself. It had a cat on it.

But when I was with my first boyfriend aged seventeen, I started to notice my boobs more. I noticed that my left one was smaller than my right. I was with a boy who couldn't give a hoot; I could have had cyclops boobs for all he cared – he adored me. But it started to bother me, and so when I noticed a mole growing on my right boob

I thought it was a good opportunity, or rather an excuse, to visit my GP and bring up the boob-size situation. This GP would end up being the same GP who a few years later would tell me my lumpy boob was 'normal'. And back then she thought my mole was normal (which it was) and the fact it was growing on a boob that was substantially larger than my other boob was totally 'normal' as well. I would discuss my asymmetrical boob woes with the boyfriend, and momentarily he'd make me feel better about it all, saying that I could do something about it if I really wanted. And I guess he was right. And if it had bothered me that much, I might have. But instead I got on with life.

Two years later I was forced to notice my boobs again, as they'd left a little orange mark on the inside of my white T-shirt bra. This, ladies and gentlemen, is known as nipple discharge, possibly the worst words in the English dictionary. And yes, it is one of the symptoms of breast cancer. And no, I did not know this at the time. And yes, when I look back now, it was really gross. I was nineteen at this point and my then boyfriend would notice it and sometimes squeeze a bit out, but not once did he suggest I get it checked out. But I guess I can't blame him, as much as I would like to. I too presumed it was normal, that this stuff happened to girls my age. But it doesn't. Girls shouldn't have bloodstained liquid coming out of their nipples, EVER. So I lived with a lopsided chest and a leaky boob for about two to three years. Yup, writing that makes me feel really foolish and really embarrassed, and yeah, throw in some shame for good measure. But, I convince myself, without someone telling you differently, how would you ever know it wasn't right!? I refuse to blame myself – mainly because, well, it wouldn't change anything, and my reality is hard enough without the guilt. It wasn't until my boob started to become painful that I thought it needed further investigation.

As all of this was going on, I was also trying to figure life out. After two years out of education and some coaxing from my mum, I had enrolled in an HND (a Higher National Diploma) in travel and tourism management at Northampton University. Towards the end of it we were given the decision to stay on for another year to get ourselves a full degree, but I didn't care about a degree. I wanted out – and fast, and since the boy I had been going out with was in China, I made it my mission to find myself a job over there, doing what I thought would be the dream – working in tourism! I scored myself an internship through a school in Beijing, which would allow me to not only work at a French–Chinese travel company and thus earn money, but also learn Mandarin too. I felt like I'd finally won at life.

Before that adventure began, my twin sister, Maren, and Mum arranged a short girls-only trip to Barcelona, as we weren't sure when I'd be back from China, and when we could next spend this kind of time together. One evening, while in our hotel room, I mentioned to them that I had a hard area on the top half of my left boob, and that it was quite painful. My toes curled telling them; this wasn't our usual topic of conversation. But maybe by telling them I could stop worrying. They would tell me to stop being silly, wouldn't they? My annoyingly larger right boob was *sans* lumpy area, so I wanted their opinion on the matter: I wanted them to tell me they had the exact same thing happening with their boobs. Instead Maren agreed it was a bit odd. Mum, ever the one to imagine worst-case scenarios, demanded I go to the GP ASAP. As much as I was disappointed that moment didn't end in them poking fun at me for, ya know, thinking a leaky, painful boob *wasn't* normal, for once I appreciated Mum insisting that I get it checked out (not that she ever voiced her worry that it could be cancer, but she may well have been thinking it). So on our return I booked an appointment to see our GP, the same one we'd been seeing for years. She examined me, asked me about my periods, then declared: 'It's probably hormonal.'

I was taking the progesterone-only 'mini-pill' at the time, which she thought could be the cause. I told her of my impending adventures in Beijing, and she thought it best not to try a new contraceptive pill before I left in case I didn't get on with it very well. I happily agreed.

Instead she recommended I take evening primrose oil to help with the tenderness. I was over the bloody moon. It was exactly what I wanted to hear. In my mind I was already in Beijing, and for anyone or anything to scupper that plan was not an option.

And off I buggered. Beijing was one of those places you would either find a fun challenge or hellishly frustrating. The people, the culture, the traffic, the bureaucracy, everything was overwhelming at times, but I loved it. I absorbed it all and engrossed myself in the life of an expat Beijinger. My boyfriend at the time was no longer in China so I was there alone, finding my feet through the friends I made at the language school. Each morning I'd fight my way onto the overcrowded metro to my office job in a high-rise overlooking buildings that had sprung up in literal days in preparation for the Olympics. At weekends, when it was guaranteed to be sunny (because the government ensured it was), I'd ride my rickety bike that I bought off a German, a fellow student from the school who'd returned home, and meander down the many little hutongs taking in the innumerable aromas that city back streets offer. I was having a real-life adventure, and although I ended up hating the internship and later quitting to teach English (and by teach, I mean repeat words over and over in the hope that they'd stick), I learned a lot, grew up a lot and started to get to know myself a little more. Some nights I noticed some discomfort when lying on my front. My left boob would sometimes even feel like it was burning up. I dutifully downed as much evening primrose oil as I could; in my head, it was helping, because the GP told me it would. When I ran out I even got Mum to send me more – I didn't risk trying to find it or an equivalent in Beijing.

I went out a lot. I lived as hedonistic a life as I could have wanted, stumbling out of nightclubs as the sun was rising. One wintery evening I went out with a couple of friends but decided to not drink, as I was already feeling a bit off. At the small bar we were standing in I started to feel horrendously faint and made the decision to head home. As soon as I got to my apartment I found myself hugging the toilet. Suddenly, as I retched, I felt something 'ping' in my lower spine. This turned me into a very slow-shuffling granny for the following two or three weeks. It didn't really ever get better, only manageable. I can remember thinking how unfortunate and unfair it was that I'd been so unwell without even drinking, and then to hurt myself as I puked! I made up for it with proper alcohol-fuelled nights as soon as my back allowed. Then Christmas time arrived and I wanted to be home. The lease on my apartment was up and so was my time at the school. My teaching jobs were non-contractual (cash in hand) so I took the opportunity to leave Beijing with a vague plan to hopefully return in the New Year, perhaps with a visa and, who knows, maybe some actual teaching qualifications.

I made an appointment with my GP as soon as I landed, as there were a few things I wanted to discuss with her, including, of course, my boob. My GP was on holiday, so I got the substitute male doctor, who I already wasn't a big fan of. I never appreciated his abruptness and uncaring tone. And this appointment was no different. The fact I knew them all so well makes it sound like I visited the GP a lot, and I suppose I did. In my early twenties I had recurring cystitis and UTIs (until I learned a pint of water after sex and flushing out my bladder would stop it from happening – it would help if they taught you such life hacks at school) that required a lot of antibiotic prescriptions. I had also suffered from headaches for as long as I could remember, so trying to get to the cause of those involved many doctors too. I mentioned to the GP that my boob lump had not got any better, and in fact was starting to feel more tender. The only response I got out of him was that I could switch my contraceptive pill if I wanted to, but that the examination I had received seven months earlier by the lady GP would suffice and was enough evidence to suggest that this was 'hormonal'. And that was it. Case closed.

On telling Mum what had happened at the surgery, her frustration turned to anger. How could he not even suggest a referral, she fumed, or at the very least examine my boob? I felt a bit silly for not pushing it more. Perhaps I'd played it down too much; perhaps Mum was right and I should have demanded a referral. I decided to make another appointment for when my own GP was back from her holiday. She'd felt my boob before, so could tell me if it had changed. Still nonchalant and unbothered by my recalling of the last seven months, she reluctantly referred me to the breast clinic at Northampton Hospital. She warned that, because I was under thirty, and thus a very non-urgent case, it could take six weeks for the appointment.

In the meantime, a New Year's family skiing trip had been arranged, which I was looking forward to – returning home from Beijing was a hard adjustment. I was in a quandary about what to do next, whether to go back to China or perhaps somewhere new, or spend some time with Maren in Cornwall while I figured out my next steps. I knew the ski trip would help keep my mind off life decisions for another week at least. We had joined up two families: ours, and Maren's boyfriend Graham's family – his dad, stepmum, brother and sister. I had never skied before, not even on a fake snow slope, but I think that was to my advantage, as I had no fear, and would just launch myself down some (admittedly pretty pathetic) little hills. There were injuries but luckily not for me, and as attention was on our invalids, no one noticed I was in the corner holding a heat pad to my lower spine and my boob. That is how bad the pain had become. Yup, I know.

On our return home a hospital letter was waiting for me, inviting me to an appointment at Northampton General Hospital's breast clinic in six weeks' time. Mum came in handy again, pushing me to call them daily to see if there were any cancellations. I managed to score myself an appointment with a consultant ten days later. As promised, my GP had referred me to the boob specialist for further examinations and presumably some tests. This was my first step on the ladder of the breast cancer system: a meeting with a consultant surgeon, not a Dr, but a Mr.

At that first appointment Mr Dawson asked me questions I was pretty much expecting: when did I notice the lump? Was there a family history of breast disease? Was I on the pill? Did I have regular periods? All my answers were a bit wishy-washy; the only thing I could say for sure was that Nanna had breast cancer at thirty, but she didn't die – in fact she only had a mastectomy, no further treatments, and went on to have kids and live a long and happy life until the age of seventy-five. He carried out an ultrasound to see the difference in substance of my two boobs, and to rule out a cyst – which would show up as a liquid. The scan confirmed that my lump was indeed a hard, non-liquid one, but before he could take this any further he wanted me to wait three weeks to see if coming off the pill would make any difference to my hormones and thus the lump. Hormones. My stupid hormones again.

I wasn't convinced. I'd had weird periods all my life, so it's not like I could say for sure whether my boobs changed with my cycle. Also I had no clue when my cycle was, that's how irregular they were. But what could I do? Stamp my feet and demand further examinations there and then? Perhaps some people might, but I didn't. And so I waited for three long weeks.

By this time my lower back had been giving me all kinds of grief. Visiting Maren in Cornwall, I decided to visit a chiropractor, a lovely lady named Helen. She treated me three times before concluding it wasn't getting any better. She was one of the good chiropractors, the ones who don't keep seeing you, not fixing you and taking your money anyway; she encouraged me to get an X-ray instead. Which I did. But the results were going to take a couple of weeks, and so my breast appointment came before the X-ray results.

This time in my life was particularly weird. It felt like life had stalled; every time I started to think about making plans to go back to China or get teaching qualifications, I felt that I was stuck until I knew what was going on with my body. To earn a little pocket money I spent some time in Cornwall life modelling (don't get too excited, with my clothes on) for art students. I felt so bad telling them after five minutes that I needed to sit down, that the pain in my back was too much.

Back home I spent a night out with one of my best friends, Lou, staying at our pal Adam's house in Milton Keynes. After a night of dancing at Oceana (name-checking it here purely so I never forget that such places existed and were part of my youth) and general silliness, Lou and I shared a bed at Adam's. Waking up, somewhat blurry that Saturday morning, I noticed a big damp patch down my front. On inspection I saw an orange liquid had obviously leaked out of my boob in the night, staining my T-shirt and, very embarrassingly, the duvet cover too. I was mortified. My boob had wet the bed! Lou called her mum, who was a nurse at the same surgery I had been going to, to get her advice. She was calm, reassured both me and Lou that it would be fine. Only recently did I discover that Lou's mum was secretly really concerned about what was happening to me, but hid it well, thinking there was no point in alarming me when I had follow-up appointments imminently. But when I got home and showed Mum my T-shirt, her anger turned to rage. 'If this ends up being worse than we think, I am thumping your GP.' Just so you know, Mum is not violent in any way, ever. She obviously didn't mean it, although I would love to have watched my mum deck a male doctor.

I didn't dare ask her what she meant by 'worse than we think'.

Along came the day of the follow-up with Mr Dawson. I told him of my night-time boob explosion; I even took the T-shirt as evidence, as by this point I didn't want anyone to convince me that this was nothing, even though I'd given very little thought to what the opposite of nothing could be. At last there seemed to be a shift. He wanted me to have a mammogram there and then, followed by a biopsy. I didn't know what any of this stuff entailed. Mum had had a couple of routine mammograms and had told me how they clamped your boobs, but nothing prepared me for the pain. Of course it hurt: not only was it crushing my breast away from my body, it was squashing what was by then a six- by nine-centimetre growth. I leaked some orange liquid onto the scanning plate; I glanced at the nurse to see her reaction, but she wore her best poker face. On the inside I was dying of embarrassment, and my face probably gave that away.

I struggled to get on to the bed for my biopsy. The gentle-voiced radiologist asked me what was wrong and I told him of my Beijing escapades and that night I puked and put my back out. He chuckled. And then proceeded to insert a giant needle into my boob with the aim of grabbing a little bit of the growth so it could be sent off for tests. He didn't manage it on the first go (it did look pretty fiddly) but after a second painful prod he was happy that he'd managed to get enough to biopsy. He was doing all of this while looking at an ultrasound screen. There I was, lying on a bed staring at a screen like an expectant mum. Only I wasn't looking lovingly at my growing baby but at a potential mutant growth. And instead of finding out the sex, we'd be waiting to hear if it was there to kill me or not.

'I can't tell you that this is nothing to worry about,' he said, candidly.

I am not sure why he felt the need to say this, but I was grateful for the honesty.

One week later I was back receiving the results in that cold, tiny, clinical consultation room.

'There are three things you need to remember from this news,' Mr Dawson said.

I remembered none of them. His voice became noise as I tried desperately to stay composed. The radiologist had told him of my struggle to get on to the bed during my biopsy and so he'd ordered some further scans to happen over the next few days, with a follow-up appointment to see him with results a week from then. He mentioned an operation to remove the lump and with it my boob. He seemed keen to do that soon. There were probably more words exchanged, but it's a blur now. I walked out of the room clasping a blue folder full of pamphlets about breast cancer, the surgery, support groups. The folder signifying my membership of a club I hadn't applied to nor wanted to be in. A members-only club whose membership fee you wouldn't want to pay even if you could afford it.

The breast cancer club.

The 'Now What?' Bit

Is there a word for knowing something to be real but not believing it? Because, *that*. I couldn't quite process what I had just been told, yet as we walked out of the hospital Mum and I were already discussing how I would be fine. How I had to be fine. I knew absolutely nothing about cancer but *It's going to be OK* became my internal mantra. We didn't know this for sure, but that didn't really matter; at that moment you fool yourself into believing anything.

'We will deal with this. It's going to be fine' were Mum's robotic, encouraging, yet very unconvincing words. But our strides to the car matched our determination. I can confidently say that I was trying to keep my shit together for my mum's sake, and I have no doubt she was doing the same for me. We were both in complete disbelief. I had just been told I had breast cancer: WHAT THE ACTUAL FUCK.

It wasn't long before I had to say the words 'I have cancer' aloud. My aunty Rosemary was staying with us, and my older sister Maike was at home during her half-term break from teaching in London. I wasn't sure what they could read from our faces; no doubt they could sense it was bad news, but not in a million years did they expect me to share the worst news possible. Their disbelief, confusion and bewilderment matched ours. And once that was out of the way, bizarrely, we stuck the kettle on and carried on the day as normal. We had planned to visit some family and so we did. We sat in my mum's aunt's living room, discussing the weather and other really important topics. But my mind was of course far, far away in a new cancer-land. I was sitting on the sofa but inside my head I was bouncing off the walls, running around in a frenzy asking WHY and WHAT and HOW over and over again, like a woman possessed.

I went to the bathroom just to escape the small talk and gather my thoughts. I stared at myself in the mirror and for the first time I didn't recognise the girl I was looking at. It was me, the outer shell of me, but somehow, inside, it really wasn't. This girl had cancer. CANCER. Mr Dawson's words raced around my head, even louder than before, as if he was screaming them in my ear. I was rerunning the scene desperately trying to reveal a different ending. That day changed everything. You might be surprised to hear that we didn't share the news with my great aunt. It didn't feel right – I guess we weren't really sure what we were dealing with at that moment, and we knew my news would be met with a bazillion questions we couldn't yet answer. Besides, I hadn't even told Maren yet, and there was no way any other family member was going to find out before her.

I met Maren in the womb. She pushed me out of our warm and cosy amniotic home seven minutes before deciding to join the party too. Mum's diary entry notes the moment Maren and I discovered each other for the first time.

Tuesday 14 January 1986: Twins discovered each other for the first time! They lay on the changing table grinning and 'talking' to each other.

Mum knew she was having twins before the scan confirmed it. She'd miscarried twin boys the year before and the advice from the direct German nurse was to forget about it and 'make more'. So she and Dad did, and it came as no surprise to her that two babies were about to come into her world. Maren and I spoke a twin language for a while. In some ways we still do. Some say when we are together our togetherness is impenetrable.

At two years old we decided to run away. I have no idea why (to this day I am convinced our older sister Maike encouraged us to). With our tiny legs we obviously didn't get far, but far enough to frighten Mum to a whole new level. Twins were a bit of a shock to Maike who, at the hospital, asked my parents which one they would be taking home. Until we came along she was the golden-locked wonder child, so it wasn't a huge surprise that she adopted the Angelica-from-*Rugrats* role whenever our parents' backs were turned. Thankfully this later blossomed into a friendlier relationship, but she would be the first to admit that the bond we have is very different from the one I have with Maren.

I love being a twin and revealing this to people at every given opportunity – it's always a really good 'super-fun fact' to use for those awful ice-breaker games. Maren and I get sad when we hear of twins who don't get along – we think it's such a waste, a waste of an egg separating inside a human body to create two more! What are the chances?! I can barely watch those shows about twins separated at birth – my emotions are too much. We once auditioned to play the part of Ruby and Garnet in the TV adaptation of Jacqueline Wilson's *Double Act*. We were not actors, but I genuinely think we believed our twin-ness would override the need to actually possess any drama skills. Needless to say we didn't get the part, *but* we did get to play extras, met loads of twins, including a pair from Scunthorpe (which I remember well because I had never met anyone from Scunthorpe before), and also got an autograph from Jacqueline herself, so, ya know.

I have appreciated being an identical twin for some

time, and it's only when I look back that I realise how lucky I was to always have someone by my side. The incessant twin questions annoy us, mainly because we can't say we are telepathic or have some freaky twin abilities. And no, Mum didn't dress us the same when we were kids, because having an older sister means you get hand-me-downs. At secondary school we did decide to get matching geeky spectacle chains. No, we didn't play tricks on boyfriends because, unsurprisingly, given the spectacle chains, we didn't have any.

And we haven't always got along. During GCSEs we decided that after sixth form we would go away for a while, to Australia. We weren't ready for university, no matter how much our grammar school wanted us to believe we were. We weren't sure what we actually wanted to study, and although I had applied for a deferred TV production course at Lancashire University, I wasn't really sure whether I actually wanted to spend any of my life studying that or, crucially, working in TV. We both needed to go and explore, grow up a little bit, and since Mum spent some time in Oz when she was a similar age, it inspired us to do the same.

We learned to cook (debatable whether you call rice, tuna and cheese cooking, but you decide), look after ourselves, be independent and budget money. We learned to be together in a whole new way and we relished it all. But on our return to the real world, and back to our boyfriends, who had waited patiently for nine months as we went off gallivanting (IKR), the gear changed and suddenly Maren and I had to find our own identities and purposes, and with that came disagreements and resentment. Boys obviously didn't help in this matter and there were some heated arguments, often about our shared Ford Fiesta. It was apparent to me that we needed to settle into our own selves and learn to appreciate each other again. Maren left to study garden design in Falmouth, in Cornwall, which helped with that. Distance made our twinship stronger, and although we suddenly saw much less of each other, we would speak on the phone often and text daily.

The text I needed to send her now, though, wasn't your usual 'How was today?' or 'OMG have you watched today's *Neighbours*?' How was I going to tell her? I texted her asking if she was in for a chat after work. She was out on a run but messaged to say she'd be back soon. I immediately texted her boyfriend Graham to make sure he would be home too when I told her, or at least not long after. All I could say is that she would need him there. By this instruction he of course knew something was up, but he didn't poke me for an explanation, he just did what he was told.

Seeing her name flash up on my phone that evening was a defining moment. I knew that once Maren heard I had cancer, I couldn't take that news back. It would also feel so much more real. I wanted to shield her from the pain, but also knew I couldn't face it without her. Once it's out there it can't be untold, and just as my life had somehow changed that day, hers would too, and for that I felt overwhelmingly guilty. That's the thing about being a twin: you live the same life in two bodies. I once had a conversation with a nosy cab driver about my illness. When he asked me how my family coped with me having the disease I said it was of course pretty hard. Especially for my twin. His response was flippant and unexpected: 'Yeah, well, it's like one heartbeat.' This floored me because I couldn't have put it better myself. Ultimately, both of us had been given a cancer diagnosis. For me in the physical sense; for her in a sense that only close twins could understand. She was about to go through every single tough day and triumph with me. Her cells might not be misbehaving, but in every other way, she was about to fight for her life, too.

It felt cruel sharing the news because I knew exactly how broken I would be if she'd ever shared news like that with me. But here's the thing: if anyone was going to get cancer out of the two of us it would be me. We were happy and mostly healthy kids and teenagers. But if anything was up, it was usually up with me. I was typically the sick one – and at age twelve I missed a lot of school due to an ongoing bout of headaches, fatigue and loss of appetite. A short stay in hospital didn't give us any answers, only that I needed to stop losing so much weight. I don't recall not eating on purpose, but I do remember thinking how much I preferred being at home to being at school. How much I loved being able to choose the food I could stomach, such as those Italian sponge fingers (also, weirdly, known as ladyfingers) instead of what my mum cooked for us. I for some reason enjoyed the attention I got that other kids didn't, like when they mentioned my name in assembly, albeit for being the sick kid who was missing a lot of school, and also the many cards my classmates wrote that Maren was sent home with to give to me.

Whether it was all part of my general growing-up issues, or whether I was in fact poorly, I still don't know now. Nevertheless, even with actual, diagnosable illnesses such as appendicitis and wisdom-tooth problems, I was first in line. So when I was diagnosed with breast cancer I never spared a moment to to question 'Why me and not Maren?' And in a sick sort of way of analysing things, we were given the right roles to adopt. Me, the invalid, who could cope with hospitals, doctors, needles and so on; Maren, the ultimate Florence Nightingale. She would be the strong one, staying calm and practical. If the tables were turned I would be a useless, helpless mess and she'd faint at the sight of needles.

I took some deep breaths. I wanted to sound strong so

she knew I was OK; from this moment she was to take her cues from me. But as soon as I heard her voice the tears rolled – so much for that bullshit. Who was I fooling? That conversation was as painful as it was life-changing. She told me she'd head home to see me as soon as she finished work the following day. 'Let's do the crying now. Crying is good. But then we crack on and deal with this, OK?' I insisted. In that moment I found some strength for the both of us, because I knew there were times ahead when that role would be reversed.

Once Maren knew, I wasn't afraid to tell others and unintentionally shit all over their days, too. It was tough each time; it was like reliving that moment at the hospital over and over again. Even recalling the words of my diagnosis now makes the hairs on my arms stand as rigidly as I did the day I heard them. But by telling people, I was rallying my troops. These were going to be the people that would keep this ship afloat, I thought, without even knowing the kind of choppy waters said ship would be sailing on and what kind of shitshow of a boat we were in. I spoke to one of my closest friends, Niall, that evening. He said, 'You beat the statistics in getting this disease at your age, so you will beat them in surviving it too.' Spoken like a true optimist. I so desperately, for once, wanted him to be right. I kept that thought in my mind, and I still do today, especially before scan results. As I did on all the calls, I tried to assure the other person I was actually all right without really knowing if I meant it, feeling some kind of obligation to sound hopeful.

Niall didn't buy it. He drove through the night, from the Highlands in Scotland to Mum's house in Northamptonshire, to check for himself that I wasn't falling to pieces. He was surprised that I wasn't a wreck. It wasn't a conscious decision not to be; absolutely nothing felt deliberate. I didn't really know how to feel, I just knew how to *do*, and what I needed to do was carry on. At first I felt bad that he'd driven 421 miles to see me, weirdly, doing OK. But what was I supposed to do? How was I supposed to react? I'm pretty sure there's no rulebook on this, no *Reacting to a Cancer Diagnosis for Dummies*. I felt numb, 'otherly', but also suddenly very held and loved. I'd not experienced such a grand and caring gesture ever before (and tbh I actually really loved it and felt I could get used to it).

Niall, Maren, Mum and I decided to take a stroll in a neighbouring town to get a change of scenery and some fresh air. You know that feeling you get when you go for a stroll in your neighbourhood or town for the first time after returning from a long holiday? Everything is very familiar, but also different; you've somehow changed. I was suddenly envious of everyone we passed in the street. How could they look so happy, so unshaken, when my world had just been so monumentally rocked?

*

The days following the news became a busy schedule of hospital tests and visits from caring friends. I had no boss to notify of my impending sick leave because, well, I was jobless. No landlord to send a note to because, well, I was back at Mum's. I was grounded, and any thought of buggering off back to China or indeed any life plans whatsoever were on hold. I was also in agony. My back pain had worsened, and by this point I couldn't stop my mind from going to scary places. Could the cancer already have spread? I didn't want to entertain that thought, and to be honest I didn't even know what that really meant but, heck, anything was possible, so how could I not think about it?

I remember so vividly my aunty coming to my room before I went to sleep and trying to reassure me that the pain was probably a completely unrelated issue. I so badly wanted to believe her, but my body and I had, for the first time in my life, started to communicate with each other – and it was telling me otherwise. I had the strongest niggle I'd ever had that I could be dealing with something far more serious, something I'd have to deal with so much longer than we might think. I smiled, nodded, was grateful that thoughts and pounding heart rates are not visible, turned the light off and somehow managed to sleep.

After having CT scans to see what else was happening in the rest of my body, along with a bone-density scan to check on my skeletal health, we headed back to the hospital one week after my initial diagnosis. This time I had full-force support in the shape of Maren, my aunty and Mum. We arrived early. We were taken to a different room, a much larger one, with more than one chair this time, but not enough for us all, so I opted to awkwardly lounge on the bed. Foresight had obviously told me to prepare for news that would leave me feeling faint and nauseous. Mr Dawson entered the room and with a soft, considered tone announced that the news wasn't great. The CT scan showed that the area in my back that had been causing me so much pain for the last three months was indeed cancer. It was not simply me 'putting my back out' that time I puked in Beijing. It was not just a sore back like so many people get. It was cancer that had got very comfy on my lumbar spine, taking up two vertebrae, which more than explained my agony.

There was sickening, echoing silence. I felt as crushed as those poor little bones. We all did. I risked a glance at Maren and saw on her face a mirror image of my own. But the thing is, I still didn't really know what all this meant, only that it wasn't particularly great. I knew that now the cancer was incurable.

Mr Dawson explained that I needed to have radiotherapy to my spine immediately, mainly to help with the pain and hopefully zap the active cancer. I understood that somehow a foot had been put on the brake. The sense of urgency, the rush to get my left boob removed the following week, was gone. When cancer has already hot-footed from the primary site (my boob) to another part in the body (my spine), it makes removing the original cancer site not the cure they originally hoped. One moment you're focused on cure, the mirage of a life *beyond* cancer, the next it's 'sustain life for as long as possible', otherwise known as palliative care.

Mr Dawson outlined the next steps, the treatment plan, the dos and don'ts – which included jumping out of a plane – but it's only now that I truly appreciate his approach to that appointment. We didn't discuss a prognosis – I didn't ask and he didn't bring it up. Instead we talked tactics and actions, treatments available now and also in the future, and it was starting my cancer 'journey' (blurgh – I hate that term) in that way that I believe determined my long-term survival. WHOA – big statement, I know, and obviously there's way more to it than that, but in not putting an end date on my life, Mr Dawson gave me permission to live. He put no expectations on my survival, and trust me, I didn't want lies, but he left the window of 'who knows' wide open. He let me breathe an air of hopeful maybes and I am so, *so* grateful for that now. He could have told me my cancer was terminal, but he didn't. I might have been terminally ill, but he let me believe that I was terminally not bloody ready to die.

Since my mastectomy was no longer happening imminently, the plan instead was for me to try some hormone treatment called Tamoxifen to shrink the tumour. Now that curing the cancer was off the table, symptom management was prioritised, quality of life was considered, and I suddenly had a very busy diary. There wasn't much else I remember from that appointment, only that my aunty broached the subject of me going to the Royal Marsden in London for a second opinion. The consultant agreed – I mean, how could he not? I had gotten into this pickle by putting faith in medical professionals, but that trust was now well and truly shattered. If I needed second, third, or more opinions to feel confident and in control of my treatment plan going forward, then so be it.

Later that day our house was livelier than usual. With both sisters now at home, my aunty and then my friend Rach coming over for the evening, there was a good amount of noise and distractions to almost silence the fear. My head was spinning. But I couldn't really understand why. Apart from my back I felt well. Nothing had changed from eight days earlier – just some slightly darker bits on a scan and some words written on paper. But I guess I was playing out the emotions and reacting to the fear I had been exposed to. I didn't personally know anyone who'd died of cancer, and I definitely didn't know anyone young with this disease, but the media conditions us to panic, conveying cancer as a terrifying killer. I mean, when did you last see a cancer story in a movie that didn't end in a sad, long, miserable death? Me neither.

I listened in on the general chit-chat the others were having, participating more with facial expressions and the odd nod than with words. They may have been just as scared as me but did their best to be 'normal' and to make sure we all ate dinner like normal, functioning people do. I didn't feel like a normal person any more. I felt a bit like an alien. A confused, sad, terrified, yet strangely optimistic alien.

I didn't know what having cancer that was incurable really meant. Not until I googled it at 2 a.m., of course – the night I stupidly tuned into I'm Going To Die FM. I mean, why wouldn't you scare yourself shitless in the middle of the night, when your life already feels like it is caving in? As soon as you type 'secondary breast cancer' and hit 'enter', you nosedive into a huge, slippery, messy black hole. And you ain't coming out. There in clear, bold letters it said: 'Average survival time two to three years.' I quickly shut my laptop and took some deep breaths. I tried to convince myself that wasn't going to be *my* reality. Statistics were just numbers. I was not a number: I was a human. A human who weirdly believed in endless possibilities (I don't know why, but I did), some new-found hope that had come from somewhere mysterious, and Niall's words: 'You beat the statistics in getting this disease at your age, so you will beat them in surviving it too.' Statistics did not give my diagnosis meaning; it would be me who would do that. The meaning was obviously unclear at that time, but I knew that I would accept it. I did not yet know that I would build my whole life around cancer and find the purest of joys from it. It was all unknown to me then as I sat on my mum's sofa trying to calm my breathing.

In my diary entry for 19 February I wrote that life had changed forever on that day. And, duh, I was right. But not just life – *I* had changed forever.

Before the Turd

The greatest hazard of all, losing one's self, can occur very quietly in the world, as if it were nothing at all. No other loss can occur so quietly; any other loss – an arm, a leg, five dollars, a wife, etc. – is sure to be noticed.

Søren Kierkegaard

When I think of Kris BC (before cancer) I hardly recognise her. She is like the friend from school you vowed you'd stay in touch with and then sort of forgot, but who still springs to mind from time to time and who you might stalk on Facebook. She was unambitious, painfully unsure of herself, dying to have a purpose but unaware what that meant. I guess she was a normal twenty-three-year-old who hadn't quite sussed life out yet, and who could blame her? Who can really say for sure, at twenty-three, what they want to become? I was always envious of and a bit puzzled by people who had got life sorted by the time they were taking their GCSEs. The ones who knew they'd be a doctor or vet annoyed me the most. How did they know? What gave them such drive? I knew nothing other than to obsess over and get through my GCSEs without really knowing why or what for. I was born into a family of teachers, with my great-grandad and grandad, and then my dad and his sister following suit, but that never seemed for me. My parents never pushed me into anything, especially anything academic; for them happiness seemed to be as good a goal as a successful career.

But what even was happiness? I was pretty certain that the 'typical' path wasn't for me – the one where you meet your soulmate, get married and have babies, that is. I couldn't be sure it would lead to said happiness or fulfil-ment and I wasn't too sure I wanted to find out, either. I was also weirdly convinced, from a really young age, that I was infertile. I can't explain why, I just was. I knew that growing up meant becoming things; I just wasn't too sure what those things were. Basically I was a bit lost, but I guess having so little pressure on me (from others or from myself) to be something has helped me to come to terms with what my life has turned out to be.

I have always hated change. I feared school trips away from home because it was so different from normal life. I was so uncomfortable with being away from home that often my mum joined us on school outings – I was *that* kid. I was born in a small town in Germany called Norden, on the North Sea coast, where the land is pancake-flat apart from the dykes that protect the land from the sea, and where they speak a weird type of German; a place I can bet you've never heard of or visited, although I do highly recommend it – off the coast there are some of the most stunning islands and beaches on the planet (who knew?). My British mum met my German dad when she was almost eighteen years old and he was a twenty-six-year-old German supply teacher visiting her school. After falling madly and stupidly in love (like you do at seventeen) she followed him to Germany, where she eventually remained, married, and gave birth to my big sister Maike and, two years later, me and my twin sister Maren.

Small Kris had a lot of energy, usually expended in building dens (or full-blown bars and eateries serving up flower soup in the garden) and hunting for four-leaf clovers in the grass. Summers seemed to go on forever back then, the smell and sight of buddleia always taking me back to those long warm days. When not outside, Maren and I would be working in our restaurant, 'Maki', which hijacked the living room, or perhaps at our pretend travel agency or divorce lawyers' office. You mean to say that you *didn't* play at creating divorce papers for your mum to sign? Maren and I had a pretty wild imagination, but not so much in the fantasy scene, more the real-world stuff. Stuff that was playing out IRL and could, I don't know, perhaps be helpful or a cheerful distraction for Mum. School was carefree. I was a classic geek who never got into any trouble, adored my teachers and obsessed over homework. I loved anything creative, always being the first absolute loser to volunteer for a fun art project.

I was a mummy's girl – if there was ever an opportunity to spend the day with our dad, I wouldn't take it, however much I was asked (but never forced) to. Apart from the odd morning at Sunday school (we were not religious) spent singing biblical songs (weird, I know) accompanied by Dad's guitar playing, I'd leave it to my sisters to spend time with Dad while I felt the need, a sense of duty, to be with Mum. I appointed myself as her protector. I remember only too well a night I had to spend at my Oma's house when I was about seven or eight. What for any other kid would seem like a fun thing to do because it involved a long summer's day playing in her big garden, dancing with teddies, scooping frogs and tadpoles out of her pond, turned into a day of tears for me. I was sad, so sad, and I couldn't really express why. Even having my twin sister with me didn't console me. I liked the comfort of home, my safe surroundings, and knowing Mum was OK. I guess my grandma, Dad and Maren figured out a way to distract me enough that I settled my tears and accepted I was to be there for the night. I wasn't a brat; I was scared. I had big feelings when I was a kid and did not know what to do with them other than to suppress them or cry a lot.

I knew from the moment I could know stuff that my mum and dad didn't like each other. I remember vividly the daily arguments around the dinner table, which resulted in Dad storming out and Mum screaming and making all sorts of hand gestures – which I then didn't understand, baffled why she would stick sometimes one, often two fingers up at the door. *Abendbrot* ('evening bread') was very often fraught with tension. I remember Mum's pained, false smiles at family events and how much she hated pretending to be a happy family. I noticed it all, perhaps too much. She was burdened by her life choices and disappointments and often had no one to lay them on but her daughters. But my parents' relationship seemed normal to me. It seemed normal to me that my mum would threaten that she'd run away from it all, that she'd leave and never come back. There were days I just knew she hated life so much and although I was too young to understand mental health and suicide, she made it feel very plausible that she might really go away somewhere and not come back.

It seemed normal that at six and seven I was waiting for my mum to come home from teaching evening school, hanging out of the bathroom window to wait for her car to pull up, crying with relief as I hugged her, breathing in the smell of the fresh, cold outdoors that clung to her hair. I probably had no concept of time or whether she was actually ever back later than she should have been, but there was no way I'd sleep if she wasn't home. The times Mum visited London with her evening-school ladies were the WORST and I missed her so much – but was always consoled by the gifts she'd bring back from the Disney Store (like those plastic beaker cups that had a layer of water inside them with floating glitter. Remember them?) Keeping Mum happy was something I took upon myself from way too young an age, when my focus should have been more on making friendship bracelets or creating hamster houses than on my mum's sanity. But I adored my mum. She was fun, creative and full of ways to make any occasion, such as a birthday or the German tradition of Carnival, exciting and action-packed.

I'm pretty sure she was solely responsible for making Halloween a thing in Germany, too – much to the joy of all my friends, who loved it every time we announced we were having yet another party. She'd hand-make us costumes for events or ballet performances, and clothes, sometimes working all night to finish them to perfection. She poured every ounce of love and care into us. Whenever she could and funds allowed, she took us on holiday to Switzerland, Canada and to England to see her family – she instilled in us all an insatiable need to travel and see the world. My dad would hardly ever join us, despite the fact that as a teacher he was off work as much as we were off school, but I never questioned it because it, again, seemed normal.

My only memories of my dad, growing up, are being carried up to bed by him some nights, him drinking German Berocca (I was obsessed with watching the tablet fizz away in his glass), his devotion to collecting all and any new electrical gadget – mainly TV, video or cameras – and his ability to turn on the charm around people that weren't his family. I recall particularly forced moments when he curiously felt the need to impress new people, such as when we met the couple from East Germany who'd found a note attached to a balloon I launched (as part of some event) who travelled to see us after the Berlin Wall came down (I was three when that happened and I sadly can't remember it). But for some reason I remember his need to show us off. He'd struggle to say it, but I knew he was proud of my school or ballet achievements. However forced or false I thought he might appear, everyone seemed to think diamonds shone out of my dad's bumhole. All his family were in complete denial about his obnoxious behaviour towards Mum and his ineptitude as a dad of three. Even when calling her own family in England, Mum didn't receive any support, instead enduring arguments about why she should stay with him as he was a 'good man'. The age-old 'man providing for family is as good as it gets' adage had not been shaken off on either side of the family. Mum found herself with someone that no one else seemed to see.

When Maren and I were nine, Mum finally had evidence that my dad was sleeping with other women (had been since we were two – I will spare you the details), and it was only then that her own mum believed her. After just one phone call to her parents, it was decided: we were finally leaving Dad and moving to England. She needed the support of her parents more than ever and it makes me sad knowing it took evidence for her family finally to accept she was desperately unhappy. I didn't need convincing, of course; I was only ever on Mum's side. Even when I mention now how I was such a mummy's girl, my mum likes to bring up this ONE time I cried for my dad.

The only reason we can all recall this time is because we have video evidence of it. To me it looks like a kid who was overtired and needed a sob, but apparently I was sad that my dad was leaving to go somewhere – I don't recall where. I was only about three, but I remember being laughed at a lot for wanting him. It was uncharacteristic of me and I guess a surprise and shock to Mum because – well, he wasn't a particularly great, loving, nurturing or even fun dad, so how could I be sad to see him go? I will never know what was actually the matter with me, and it's irrelevant now. What I find strange is how everyone, even my sisters, mocked me for wanting my dad, and in doing so it made me feel that wasn't OK.

Mum waited until Maren and I had finished junior school before making the big move to England. It was the biggest adjustment of my life – before cancer trumped that, of course. It took a more grown-up brain and perspective to really appreciate and respect Mum's huge strength to move three children to another country and uproot not only their young lives but hers too, giving up the entire life she had built for herself since she was seventeen. Looking after us on her own wasn't new to her, though, as she felt she'd done that since day dot.

I didn't feel in the slightest bit sad that I'd barely see my dad any more. It was the change of location, having to wear a school uniform (not a thing in Germany), living with my grandparents, sharing a bed with my sisters, that had the biggest impact on me. Maren and I were put in the same Year 6 class at primary school and because our English was so embarrassing we refused to speak anything but German or Twinnish with each other, which, I can tell you, is not the best way to make friends. I cried and cried. I cried in secret in the school toilets and I cried myself to sleep. I cried so much that I think it became sort of normal at dinner, and as I sobbed into my food, my sisters, grandparents and Mum would carry out normal catch-ups on the days they had had. I couldn't work out or explain why

I was so sad, only that I didn't like all the change. All this injustice and grief had built up in me and the reassuring and familiar confidence I felt in German life was stifled. I didn't miss anything specific about Germany; I just hated not knowing or recognising anything about this new life.

The day Maren was unwell and couldn't go to school with me was the first worst of my life. I couldn't understand how I could possibly survive the day, endure conversations with the other kids, understand my schoolwork, eat at lunch without her.

It feels like that transition to acceptance took forever, but remember I was just ten, and stuff that probably only affected me for five minutes felt like eternity then and even now. I don't remember the day it got easier, but it must have happened because, well, it had to. I had no choice but to keep going to school, speak English in the playground so we could play with our classmates – our first ever English friend, Faye, thought our Germanness was more fascinating than weird – and eat my cream-cheese-and-cucumber sandwiches at lunchtime (in Germany we'd be back home for lunch with Mum by 1 p.m.). And eventually, especially when the four of us had our own home, I was OK. The tears stopped, I took a deep breath and suddenly it became my new normal.

Eventually I became a kid who was actually more English than German – although it took some time to shake the accent. Even now a German word will pop into my head from time to time. I think there are certain -isms of a language you can never unlearn. It was an early lesson in acceptance, bigger than having to accept *Neighbours* moving from BBC to Channel 5, but maybe not quite as big as cancer.

I think starting a whole new life aged ten was the first time I learned how to accept the unshakable truth that life can change dramatically. I had no choice in the matter: I mean, who has any sort of control of their life at the age of ten? I was a kid who lacked power and agency over anything much. I was what I thought I needed to be at that time: a good girl, a good daughter, a good student. I knew what I needed to be, but not *who* I wanted to be. I didn't argue about the move, in fact I don't remember stringing any words together about how I actually felt, other than telling a divorce solicitor that I of course wanted to live with Mum; I don't recall ever imagining an alternative. I knew I had to be strong even when I really, *really* didn't want to be. Ten-year-old Kris didn't know those very same feelings would be smacking her round the chops thirteen years later.

Boys

You have to kiss a few frogs.

My nanna Vera

I was seventeen when I first ventured into a relationship with a boy. I say ventured, but it was in fact a massive leap. Puberty-stricken me wasn't even interested in the very existence of boys, let alone being in a relationship with one. I was a late bloomer in every sense – I started my periods when I was fifteen! Is it possible to be so in denial about the inevitable that your body holds off until the very last moment? In my head my ovaries would hold AGMs about whether I was ready and decide I very much wasn't. Until of course they couldn't hold out any longer. And then it happened. During a drama lesson at school. I wanted to die.

Anyway, Maren and I were far too busy being 'boffs' – taking school projects very seriously (you should have seen the miniature Tempest Island we built!); making up dances; recreating sketches from our favourite show, *Smack the Pony*, with our friend Faye; directing music videos; or playing with our guinea pig and hamster friends – to entertain the idea that we could, I dunno, spend time with boys. I mean, of course I dabbled in talking to boys in random online chat rooms like ICQ, convincing some Canadian ones we were older than we were (so much so that I put a '16' in my Hotmail email account to make it more obvious and factual – sweetychick16@hotmail.com). And then, as sudden as lightning, I fell fully and deeply in love with my first real-life love, having never experienced even so much as a crush on someone before – no posters of male pop stars ever hung on our shared bedroom wall, just polar bears and penguins, because polar bears are great.

He was a local boy I eyed up every time Maren, our friend Beth and I hung out at the rec (recreation ground, for those not familiar with cool places for teenagers to hang). We would ever so casually pretend we were there to swing on the swings, but would very obviously fool around for attention while he and his friends rode their BMX bikes on the ramps. By fool around I don't mean setting light to stuff or sharing fags behind a bike shed, I mean swinging as high as possible and kicking our legs out to send our shoes flying off our feet – the winner was the one who could toss them the furthest. We wanted them to notice us. I wanted Sam to notice me. I blushed whenever he so much as looked at me. His smile melted me into goo, as did his strong arms, which he flexed doing tricks on his bike. I wore Etnies skater shoes to impress him but have still to this day not stepped on a skateboard. He had gone to the rival school in our town but we had mutual friends, and so through them I had reliable information that he wasn't a bully, didn't get into trouble much (but also wasn't a loser) and had friends and a car – all necessary attributes to me.

Once Sam and I finally spent time together and chatted nightly on MSN, he sheepishly asked me to be his girlfriend (via a text that I sneakily read when dipping into the cutlery and crockery cupboard at my hotel waitressing job). I swiftly forgot what life without a boyfriend was like. I romantically and unceremoniously lost my virginity to him in a tent and it was every bit as awful and awkward as your first time is meant to be. (Slightly off-topic, but isn't it weird that we say 'lost'? Like I misplaced my wallet.) Being with him was intense and full on, and we were inseparable for about eighteen months, but then, after school, it was time for me and Maren to go exploring and work our way around Australia. Sam and I didn't really discuss breaking up and he offered to wait for me and *man* I cried saying goodbye to him at the airport. But a plan was a plan.

Hindsight has me pondering whether staying in a relationship while you go travelling aged eighteen is a good idea (conclusion: it's not). I was having new experiences and changed a lot in that time, but he was back at home living out life in the same job, with the same friends, smoking too much weed – the same small-town routine, day in, day out. Yes, this caused unfair friction and, naturally, when I got home I got twitchy and restless because the poor bugger hadn't experienced what I had. Still, what that relationship taught me is that boys can be ever so nice and caring and truthful, and I feel lucky I started my journey into grown-up-hood with a decent human being. Cute.

But when I was nineteen I decided sweet, caring and truthful was easily substituted with something a bit more unpredictable, cheeky and wild – in other words, heart-breaking and hard work. I met a boy that would end up undoing all the faith and security I had built up from my first fairly innocuous relationship – but who wants innoc-uous? No Sherlock is needed to work out that my second ever relationship mirrored my parents' – he the charmer, me the rabbit in the headlights, waiting for my fragile self-worth to be run over. Just imagine the type of guy Lizzo sings about and that should paint an accurate picture. Let's call him Dan. That's not his name, but I ought to protect his identity. Am I too nice? I'm too nice.

Dan and I met at an age when neither of us knew what life could really offer and what we could grab from it. I was driving myself and my family crazy swivelling between starting a degree, then not, then deciding maybe

I should be an easyJet hostess and even going for an interview in Luton, before deciding the daily cabin pressure wouldn't work well with my frequent headaches, and then booking an impromptu month-long volunteering trip to look after some orangutans in Borneo. I sounded hella independent, didn't I? On the outside I was; internally my focus was always on others, and, soon, on Dan. Even in the depths of the fuck-knows-somewhere rainforest, I was wondering whether he would call. Whether he was missing me. I don't really know why I bothered going away when my head was always somewhere else. Of course I enjoyed my time in Borneo and *sure* I bonded with an orangutan called Doris, got chased by a protective mother ape, eaten alive by leeches and had the best time with a girl called Louise who, like me, expected there to be a big group of volunteers only to find, to our horror, that it was just the two of us working in the middle of a rainforest with sanctuary staff who spoke very little English. I loved the adventure, I loved the independence and the confidence I grew, but I always seemed to need that reassurance that someone was waiting for me at home. Dan capitalised on that vulnerability by telling me how important I was, how much he'd be lost without me and then failing to respond to messages or calls. He spoon-fed me crumbs of interaction that made me think I needed him to validate my very existence.

The same year I was struggling with life indecisions was also the year my dad died unexpectedly. Dan was there for me. But it's possible to be there, but not really *there*, ya know? I needed words, comfort, distractions and the opportunity to express all my muddled feelings, even if they made no sense at all. In fact, the first time Dan told me he loved me was shortly before my dad's funeral. Am I a bitch or is that not AT ALL useful in that moment? Dan didn't really say or do anything that made me feel particularly better, because he didn't have the emotional maturity to do so.

After Dad's death I spent some time at our house in Germany, where Dad had stayed after he and my mum divorced. As he hadn't written a will and had hoarded too much stuff, it became my job (as my sisters were at uni or working) and Mum's arse-ache to pick up the pieces and clear his house before selling it. I didn't know how to handle that situation at all. I was struggling to grieve the death of a father I wasn't sure I really liked all that much. After our move I spoke to Dad on the phone fairly often, and Maren and I received a joint card from him for our birthday each year. I saw him about once or twice a year, when we'd either head back to Germany (in a car packed to the rafters with salt and vinegar Walkers crisps, cheddar cheese, Branston pickle, Cadbury's chocolate, all his British faves) or he'd visit us in the summer holidays. I don't remember ever being excited at the prospect of seeing him. But now I was bothered by how suddenly he'd died, without warning, and how I would never have the opportunity to try and understand him. Grief is a multifaceted beast that I didn't have the brain power or capacity to slay.

Dan's empty words were a temporary plaster, and his neediness at least filled some time. He was also a musician and so of course he would send me recordings of his latest material. 'I'm really struggling today,' I'd say. Probably over MSN or MySpace.

'Ah man, that sucks. Did you listen to the track I sent?' he'd reply.

And of course I would tell him how wonderful it all was. (You wouldn't have heard of him because he, well, unlike Lizzo, didn't hit the big time.)

After months of deliberating I decided to do the HND in travel and tourism (it was as much of a doss as it sounds, but much like all academia, I took it seriously and was satisfied with nothing but the best grades). Life for me had more of a routine than just hanging out at Dan's parents' house eating two-minute noodles or Greggs' tuna and cucumber baguettes (drool) and watching cartoons. I was trying to get a qualification that would allow me to get paid while I travelled the world. Dan, who was doing the odd bar shift at local pubs, felt stuck – he hated our home town and repeatedly told me he needed to escape. I wasn't a fan of it either, but it hurt me to hear him say his life was shit when he had me. I was the sole confidante to his inner misery.

It was around this time that I got into the habit of going to the gym and not really eating enough. Dan didn't have to tell me to lose weight or be more toned – it was something I told myself in fear of losing him or not being good enough. I'd never considered how I felt about my body before I met him, yet suddenly I noticed how clothes hung on me, how lanky my arms were and how untoned my bum was. In a bid to be worthy of his attention and affection, I trained myself to exhaustion and focused on stupid weight loss to the point where I'd feel bad for eating more than two slices of Ryvita and an apple at lunch. It has only been in recent years that my family have admitted how concerned they were for me at that time. They are convinced I smelled like pear drops, a telltale sign that your body is in ketosis and, in other words, starving itself. I was obsessed with how my body looked, never how it felt. I wonder sometimes if it was this apathy towards my body that had me ignoring it when it was screaming for help. My brain and body connection was always intercepted by ugly thoughts.

The self-loathing was fuelled by constant paranoia. I would wake in the night and seize the opportunity to read Dan's phone, knowing that I would read texts from other girls that would break my heart. And still I stayed. Still I let his words convince me that I was something special to him. It became addictive. I didn't have much of a benchmark or reference for a healthy, loving relationship and although I can't blame my parents for showing me how horrific two people can be to each other, I don't think it helped. Had my mum not stayed with my dad with the full knowledge he had been cheating on her since I was two years old, perhaps I'd know how to avoid believing bullshit. Perhaps I wouldn't have believed Dan when he told me I couldn't live without him.

By this stage my body was already trying to tell me something my mind had tried to ignore: that I was very, very unhappy. Every bone, cell, inch of skin clammed up whenever we had sex, making it really painful, but not once did I realise it was the constant deceit and now blatant mind-fuckery from him that caused it. After a trip to a local sexual-health clinic, a doctor advised me to see a counsellor from Relate. Relate. At age twenty-one. Let that sink in a minute. I did as advised and found myself sitting on a big leather sofa telling a nice woman how the guy I was with would often make me feel really worthless with some casual verbal abuse. I didn't recognise it at the time, and I think writing this book has really let me understand how his manipulation affected me. I now applaud how hard the counsellor tried to make me see the connection between my emotions and the fact my body was saying 'nuh uh, hunny' whenever he was making the moves to initiate sex. But I was having none of it. The day the counsellor told me, in no uncertain terms, that the only real solution she could see was for me to leave him was the day I decided I did not need her. My delusions clouded everything.

Eventually Dan moved to China to pursue whatever job he could find. He had a chiselled enough face to score himself a modelling contract, which of course fed his narcissism. As soon as I completed the HND, I managed to blag myself that internship in China so I could be with him, but by the time I got to Beijing, he had to leave the country to renew his visa. It was during the Olympics and therefore getting visas was particularly difficult, as the Chinese government was determined people wouldn't outstay their welcome. But knowing he wouldn't be there didn't stop me. I had literally no other option but to finally see something through. I was terrified but excited to learn Mandarin and perhaps discover something I loved doing. Half of me wanted to believe that distance and independence would make us want each other more, the other half hoped I'd realise life was better without him. Alas, it only made my obsession stronger – not helped by the constant stream of messages telling me he loved me and missed me, of course, forever keeping a sense of control over my life.

Nonetheless, I got stuck in to work, made friends, tried my hardest to be the grown-up and independent Kris I had imagined I could be. My determination to feel like I finally knew what I was doing with my life was often fuelled by having a twin who already seemed so sorted. It was oddly reassuring and infuriating in equal measure. I envied the life Maren had forged for herself in Cornwall, the way she had smashed her uni degree and got recruited to do a landscape design job straight away, living with her lovely, financially stable, and not at all needy boyfriend, and just her general ability to appear so 'together'. To this day I am not sure if she ever actually felt that way, or if it was merely a great image she wanted me and others to see, but it was convincing enough for me to fool myself into thinking I was OK too, and made me hesitant to admit to her that I really, really wasn't.

Dan, meanwhile, had moved to Thailand to sit out the visa situation and spend time on his Thai mother's paradise island – an island we had visited the year before, when life seemed simpler. Eventually I too had to do a visa run out of China, since they only allowed shortened visits at the time, in order to continue living there. I can't tell you how much stress it was jumping the bureaucratic hoops and the sweat I sweated to sort it – so a short trip to paradise made sense, if only for the free accommodation. At least, that's the lie I fed myself and my family. It meant Dan and I could be reunited and pick up where we'd left off. Lol. It seemed so simple. In my head I managed to lock away the pain I'd already experienced. We did indeed pick up where we left off – with the same lies and the same deceit and the same amount of convincing that I was the one and only, when I had proof I wasn't.

One day I found an empty condom packet in his washbag and I asked him about it. He said – *breathe* – that it was his brother's and he really liked the design on the packaging so wanted to keep it. Yeah. Ummmm. And what did I do next? I decided that us heading back to Beijing together was a great idea so we could actually live together in a city we were now accustomed to, living in an apartment with friends I had made. 'Making it work' became my only mission. I was so desperate for an idyllic existence that I fooled my brain into thinking it was possible. And to some extent it was. We showed each other places we'd discovered during the months we'd spent there independently. Some days we were still the young, naive nineteen-year-olds that got up to stuff without consequence until, of course, I felt overwhelmed with doubts. The day I asked for his laptop password – and he gave it to me, no problem – was the day I discovered just how much betrayal you can physically feel. I was confronted with emails and Facebook messages to other girls he had slept with, saying derogatory things about me, pitying me, telling others he didn't have a girlfriend, that I did not exist. He could have said no when I asked for the password, but I think in a way he knew he couldn't hide any more; there was nowhere left to run. It was his cowardly way of admitting to the constant lying and deceit without having to open his mouth.

Everything I read shouldn't have come as a surprise to me; I had already imagined it all a million times over. It's just that I now had proof and, man, in all its black-and-white realness it was still hard to believe. I couldn't unsee the truth, and it hurt. I cried so much I ran out of tears, and absolutely nothing my flatmate Aya said or did consoled me, not even the chocolate-filled jiaozi we bought from the supermarket downstairs after a night out, nor the bottles of whisky I drank, stolen off the VIP tables in the nightclub we frequented. I fell into a deep sadness that I tried to hide and cover up as much as possible. I felt ashamed to be sad about breaking up with someone who was clearly awful, when I should have felt some relief, and I was embarrassed to still love someone who so clearly did not love me.

Maren and Mum decided to visit me just as a mild autumn turned into the icy-cold Chinese winter I'd been warned about. I mustered some excitement to show them round the world I had made for myself, show off my Mandarin (by that point I could speak to a cab driver without purely relying on hand gestures) and take them to all my favourite restaurants. But the shame never left me. All my actions and feelings were obscured by thoughts of Dan and how I could have been so dumb to trust him. The heartbreak hung like a silent veil on every thought and I couldn't escape it. I am ashamed to say that, once they went home, I let him explain himself. Yet again I tried to believe him when he said he was sorry and that he would change; that I was important enough to change for.

It was nearing Christmas and I was due to return home for a visit. Dan so nearly persuaded me not to. At home I was a sad heap of self-absorbed nothingness. Directionless, heartbroken and really quite pathetic. Even on our family skiing trip in Morzine I was berating myself for the time I had spent thinking about him, and yet, as the clock was almost striking twelve on New Year's Eve, fuelled with Prosecco and thoughtless abandon, I made a desperate call to him from the bathroom, keeping ever so quiet so the others wouldn't know what I was doing, because, of course, I had not let on that I was still in contact with him. And guess what – he didn't answer.

GUYS, I didn't think highly enough of myself to know I deserved better and that I was still being lied to. I had taught myself that the pain would be temporary and that despite everything he did and how he made me feel, that it was, in part, my problem. He would so easily judge me by his own standards, make me question my honesty and commitment, when it was him who was being the cheat and the liar. I had never learned to trust myself or believe my own feelings; I truly did not know how to. Like a puppeteer, he controlled my every move, fuelled by every single 'but I love you', 'but I need you'. I was a sucker for it. The co-dependence festered between us. It was only when something far more earth-shattering than him waltzed into my life that I realised he had manipulated and broken down every inch of the Kris I knew and thought I liked and respected. Enter stage left: cancer. The ultimate cock-block, but a life-salvaging one.

Of course, no epiphany automatically hit me as I heard the words 'you have cancer'; I needed to jump through a few more hoops and cry a few more tears before I was granted some release.

The day I was told my cancer had already spread to my spine, I got a call from Dan's parents saying they'd flown him over from China (did I mention his parents were far too good to him and that he never had money? Yeah I know, such a catch). Fighting back the tears, his mum said he was on his way to my house to see me. On the day I found out the worst news imaginable did I really want to have to deal with the emotional ballbag that was my sort-of-ex-boyfriend? No, I did not. Was I curious to know what words he could possibly string together to make me feel remotely better? Abso-fucking-lutely. Cancer may have mutated some healthy cells in my body, but it hadn't yet taken over the brain cells that made me do dumb shit. And so I allowed him to see me at my most vulnerable and most afraid. I sat in his car, like we did as carefree nineteen-year-olds, and I waited for him to soothe this ginormous wound. I waited for the comfort that I had craved since the day I met him and never saw evidence of. The same craving I had when my dad died. In my absolute desperation and delusion I needed to know whether me being terminally ill would finally make him change and step up.

None of the above surfaced. To plug a hole, I did what I had always done: allowed him to fool me into thinking he cared when I knew he didn't. But in knowing this, I could feed the self-torture that I had become so accustomed to and so in need of. For a moment I allowed my heart to be warmed, and it wasn't until he told me it was all his fault, that by hurting me he had caused my cancer, that the penny finally, *finally* dropped. In my weakest, most terrified hour, he made it about HIM. Not only had he claimed every ounce of my soul, every emotion and every thought I had about myself, he now also wanted to claim the cancer in my body: a true megalomaniac. Although I wanted to wish every bad thing that ever happened on Planet Earth on him, I didn't want to give him the satisfaction of claiming this part of me too. (Don't worry, later on I cover how he may have, in fact, been right.)

*

Ten days after arriving back in the UK to 'be with me', he finally did the best thing he could have done. He told me he was leaving to go back to China without any plan for when he was coming back. He showed me how much he cared by walking out of my life just when I needed him most. He left me suspended between an old version of myself and one I didn't know yet. And I never saw him again – until of course the universe, that minx, decided it was ready for me to, four years later, on the Piccadilly line, travelling home from Charing Cross Hospital. Every girl imagines that moment they might see their ex again, don't they? We all hope to look like we're not dying from cancer, with good hair, face on fleek, etc., but ya know what? All that didn't matter. The fact that I was childishly clasping my pink scooter didn't matter. What mattered is that he saw me well and truly living, breathing, existing without him. The hurt was gone. The anger was gone. The trust in myself felt very real and unencumbered. I almost wanted to thank him – is that weird? I felt nothing but calm. He, on the other hand, looked like he'd seen the ghost of Christmas past. It was glorious.

Should it have taken cancer for me to be free of him? No. But I didn't have the strength, self-belief, self-trust, or self-anything; in fact, I needed to know better and let go. Cancer, time, distractions challenged and changed all that. It's like it came knocking on my door and said, 'Hey, there is a life meant for you truer than the one you are living, but you have to deal with cancer in order to have it. Good luck, babes!' I finally had the freedom to *feel*, and completely on my own terms.

Of course I continued to struggle with immeasurable sadness and pain and loneliness long after he left, but there is nothing more sobering to focus on than survival. I could observe the pain from some new distance. Whether it's cancer, as in my case, or children and under-standing parents in Mum's case, I know that to be free from the chains of a toxic relationship also takes some almighty fucking strength. The day I stopped thinking about him, I knew I'd never be in a relationship that required me to abandon myself again. I realised I could mean something without belonging to someone. That I could finally trust my own thoughts and feelings. The voice I heard and could listen to that day was finally my own, and she was saying, 'Here I am, I'm taking over now.'

Apparently, I needed cancer to steer me in a direction of love and respect for myself, and believe me when I say that you cannot love what you're ashamed of.

Getting to Know the Turd

There is no such thing as a dying person; there are living people and there are dead people, and as long as somebody is alive, as long as they have any sentience or any sense about them, you have to expect and allow them to be who they have always been . . . and who they always were.

Elizabeth Gilbert, The Moth[*]

I returned to my original GP to ask for something to help me sleep. During the days following my diagnosis, Mum would sleep in my bed, stroking my head as I cried myself to delirium. Daytimes were for action and doing, but night-times offered no relief from the enormity of it all. I knew I needed help to calm my brain and saw it as an opportunity, or maybe an excuse, to see the GP who had

---

[*] Elizabeth Gilbert, *The Moth*, 18 February 2019, https://www.youtube.com/watch?v=DzH7I4usKeE

nine months earlier told me my lump was 'normal'. Maren and Mum came with me to the appointment. I think they needed her to feel the gigantic disappointment, anger and sadness that was drowning us all. We waited for an apology, some kind of acknowledgement that never came. I so badly wanted for her to at least say she could have acted differently, that she wished she'd referred me the very first time I had come to see her, but in doing so she would have to be truly human. I never saw her again after that. Today I have to live with knowing that my initial GP appointment should have happened sooner and that the conversation should have gone a bit like this:

Kris: 'My tit hurts and it's lumpy.'

GP: 'It's probably hormonal.'

Kris: 'Yup. Probably. But this isn't normal for me. This lump has been here for over two months, and I know because I check my boobs. I need a referral to the breast clinic. Stat.'

OK, maybe with less attitude. But what use is that to me now? None. I briefly looked into whether I might have a case to sue my GP, but we soon worked out that there was no way we could prove negligence. We'd need to know for sure that during those eight months I was told it was 'nothing', the cancer decided to spread to my spine. We can all guess it did, but we have no evidence. There are a lot of 'I wish' moments. Countless 'if only's.

But they provide me with no different present or future. They'd only drive me crazy. I wasn't prepared to do crazy. Anger, I decided, wouldn't necessarily be that useful either, unless I took advantage of it. I think we are too often led to believe that anger is a bad emotion, but to me, at that time, it wasn't. After all, pissed-off women make change.

Sleeplessness did not help the increasing pain in my back. Perhaps it was knowing I had tumours sitting on my spine that suddenly made the pain worse, or perhaps things were gradually progressing – but either way I needed treatment immediately.

The plan was to have five days of intensive radiotherapy to the three vertebrae that they could see were housing cancer cells. The unfortunate thing about treating the lower spine is that the beams will hit not just the cancer but anything that is in the way, in this case my bowels. After the first go I just managed to get home in time before I vomited, profusely. I was so sick we called an ambulance in a panic, as I had also broken out into hives. They didn't take me to hospital, as the nausea subsided. The subsequent treatment days became a carefully planned and timed manoeuvre because, like clockwork, my breakfast would appear precisely thirty minutes after the treatment. Anyone who has ever travelled with me, anywhere – could just be to the shops and back – will know I like to carry a sick bag wherever I go; it was the same even before cancer. A frankly brilliant trick (that has got me out of taxi-cleaning fines on several occasions) our mother passed on to us all. These have come in so handy for surprise treatment-induced nausea. This was one such occasion.

My oncologist wasn't advocating chemotherapy alongside the radiotherapy. He thought that trying the hormone treatment (since my cancer was the most hormone sensitive it could be) Tamoxifen for a while would be a good tactic before any decisions about surgery were made. I listened and considered everything he told me, but my family and I had already decided, given my journey to a very late-stage diagnosis, I should get a second opinion from what we had heard was the cancer mecca: the Royal Marsden in London. Some pals of mine had found the details of the secretary of the breast cancer oncologist, who was happy to arrange an appointment once they received a referral from my hospital with all the scans and most up-to-date reports. I felt bad at this point: I felt bad for not trusting that my oncologist had a sufficient plan in place. I felt like I was doing the dirty on my hospital when they were also providing me with good care. But here's what I say to that now, and something I wish someone had said to me then: BOLLOCKS TO FEELING BAD. Why should guilt ever come into play when you are facing a life-threatening illness? 'It shouldn't' is the answer.

The arrangements were made and an appointment soon followed, and it just so happened to be in the middle of my radiotherapy stint. Maren's boyfriend Graham drove us all – Mum, Maren and me – to London, and fuck a duck, do I remember that car journey well. Every pothole made me wince in pain, every sharp corner felt like a serrated knife carving into my back. I really needed the appointment to be worth all this agony. Once we found our way to the right department we were told that the wonder doctor had laryngitis so, although he was there, he couldn't speak, so instead I would be seeing one of his registrars. We were huddled into a consultation room.

I already anticipated what the doctor would say. I had a feeling they'd disagree with my hospital and go for a more aggressive approach. The nice lady registrar told me that, given my youth and fitness and general good health (weird thing to say when you have cancer, I know!), they strongly suggested I start a course of chemotherapy as soon as I had finished the palliative radiotherapy to my spine. She talked to us about a well-known concoction called FEC-T. She must have given some details about it all and their rationale, but all I really remember was trying to let the words 'you will lose all your hair' sink in. Despite my little to no knowledge I always assumed cancer and no hair went hand in hand.

Still, something was telling me that the aggressive approach was the one for me. I knew I could handle it, or at least wanted to give it a try. The Royal Marsden shared their suggestions with my oncologist and arrangements for a chemotherapy schedule were made – four rounds of FEC (5-fluorouracil, also known as 5-FU, epirubicin and cyclophosphamide), four rounds of T (Taxotere), all conducted at my own hospital in Northampton. Five months in total. A summer's worth of bad-cell and good-cell obliteration. Easy. As well as my chemo drugs, I'd be having a bisphosphonate IV every cycle to strengthen my bones.

An aggressive approach and one I was now aware (thanks to yet more googling) would render me infertile. Perhaps not an overly important factor when you're dealing with a deadly disease but one I still felt needed addressing, since (perhaps unsurprising as my entire medical team were blokes) it hadn't been broached and I wanted someone to talk this through with me. Naivety aside, I asked to speak to my oncologist on the phone. He seemed perplexed that I even brought it up. His response was, 'Who is to say you would be around in ten years, time to see them grow up?' There was my answer. I had half suspected that the reason they hadn't suggested egg-sparing treatments ahead of chemo was because my life was now limited, and time was of the essence, but something self-torturing needed to hear it. Thing is, I wasn't even bothered about having children, never have been (perhaps I'm lucky?). But that's beside the point. Had I been bothered, this conversation may have broken me entirely. And I think of all the women (and their partners) who have imagined children in their futures being dealt with with the same attitude, and my heart breaks on their behalf.

BLOG POST, 1 APRIL 2009

*APRIL FOOL!! You don't really have kancer ...
no? Oh, OK ...*
   Round one of chemo juice.
   Kris 1, Cancer 0.

Two weeks and one day after my first round of chemo and it was time. My hair follicles gave up the fight and decided I should adopt a new look. A time for me to discover just how many moles I have on my scalp and, best of all, to realise just how amazing head massages are with no hair. Now, I know that won't make you rush to go for the snip snip zzzzzzzzzzzz, but I wasn't half as horrified by the new look as I thought I would be.

   Before it was time to whip off my twenty-three years of hair growth, it was seriously getting annoying. I didn't have much warning – no sore scalp, no itchy-scratchiness – just hair here, there and everywhere. I left a hair murder scene wherever I went and I couldn't brush it/wash it/love it, and so covered it up every day. So during my chill-out session in beautiful Glencoe in Scotland, one very sunny evening, Niall became Mr Hair Removal Man. He took a brush to it and it kept coming and coming . . . Advice to anyone reading this, perhaps reaching this stage of treatment: sit yourself in front of a beautiful sunset and take ridiculous photos of your new 'do' at different stages of transformation. And laugh. Laugh lots. Believe me, it softens the blow. Hugs help too.

Chemo hasn't eaten my eyebrows yet, but I will keep you all updated on that.

The hair thing wasn't as bad as I had imagined. I say *imagined*, but what I mean is the conclusions I drew from movies and TV shows and societal notions were that hair = femininity. Hair loss is given a lot of negative focus whenever cancer is talked about, but for me it became part of the healing process. It was a hoop to be jumped through to get me to the next step – the next step being, at worst, not dead; at best, very well. I told myself repeatedly that the hair loss was a side effect of the treatment, the treatment that would make me better, not the cancer. That helped. The only thing that troubled me was how I was about to be perceived by the people closest to me. Stepping on the train to Scotland to spend time with Niall in the Highlands, I knew I'd be returning looking very different. I had said goodbye to my mum at the station looking like Kris, and would return looking like a cancer patient. I wasn't sure if she, or I, was ready. But how can you ever be ready?

To help, the hospital had offered me a wig-fitting appointment that involved an afternoon in a tiny room full of plastic heads with mono-emotion faces and weird contrived laughter (from me and Mum, not the heads). I thought I'd use the opportunity to have long, darker hair because, HECK, WHY NOT? I would never achieve that naturally. Sure, I could have dyed my own hair to any colour, but I'd never been brave enough and my hair never had the strength or stamina to grow very long – I didn't even have hair until I was about two years old! So I thought, *Fuck it – now is the time to live a little* (?), so I settled on a long brown wig that at first I experimented and played with using cute scarves to hide the plasticky parting – being NHS, it really wasn't that true to life. I would play 'spot the wig' when I was bored in the oncologist's waiting room, that's how crap they were. I persisted for a bit before getting so bored of actually having to look after it. The one massive perk of not having hair (aside from head massages, of course) is not having to wash it, dry it, brush it, etc., and there I was, combing fake hair. Nah. Sod that. Summer then also got so warm that I ditched it entirely, relegated it to the corner of my room, perched on top of the didgeridoo I schlepped back from Australia (because who would believe that I'd spent a gap year there had I not?), where it stayed until I realised that one whiff of it made my brain revisit smells from the hospital kitchen and chemo nausea and therefore I had to get rid.

RIP wig. RIP long (fake) hair.

I Made a Scarf

12 APRIL 2009

Hiiiiiiiiiii hombres!!

So, most of you are now aware of my bursting desire to raise awareness of young women's breast cancer and for young chicks to feel empowered to demand some action from doctors if they have any reason at all to be worried.

Anyway, I need all of you wonderfully creative/ intelligent/fabulous bods to put your bestest thinking caps on for campaign ideas and inspiration! This is why I'm having the meeting on Monday at our place for us to brainstorm and bring ideas to the table. I want it to be HUGE . . .

Basically, I'd like you to think of:

– contacts you may have – journalists/media people/campaigners

- *creative ideas, such as designs for merchandise*
- *slogans/names*
- *events and activities for an awareness week*
- *how we can spread the word.*

I appreciate any thought you give to this and totally understand if you're completely snowed under with uni work or work work or life OR you think noooooooooo thanks . . . it's cool . . . but I've selected you elite folk for a reason.

HAPPY EASTER everyone and I'll see some of you on Monday at 12 p.m. if that suits.

love love, peas and carrots
Kris x

PS. If anyone is feeling a bit ill or think they might be catching a cold please don't come on Monday, and I say that in the nicest way possible!!!!!! My immune system is at its shittiest right now and I can't take the risk . . .

In the weeks following my diagnosis, friends overwhelmed me with gifts and cards, ranging from home-made muffins sent in the post to a massive box of Sanctuary products. Everyone wanted a way to help and I wanted to give them something to feel like they were, so they felt less bad. Which, if you think about it, is actually a bit fucked up. Why are we so relentlessly solution-focused? Why don't we know that by indulging our need to 'do' and 'fix' we stifle someone's breathing space? Unless someone had in their possession the cure for cancer and wasn't telling me, I didn't need them to feel bad for not saying or doing the right thing; it was enough just to sit with me and talk to me about their lives.

I was petrified friends would start hiding what they would think were their really mundane and insignificant (in comparison to cancer) woes from me. I mean, I was desperate to hear about stuff that could take my mind off cancer. *Please indulge me in your boy troubles and period pains*, I thought. If you'd asked me what kind of person you need around you at that time, it would be spirit-lifters, not mood-hoovers.

The good thing about my pals is that they soon sensed that I didn't want to sit around talking about my shit predicament. Even on days where, yes, I probably looked like I needed to sleep, it was pointless telling me to rest: being ill only made me want to feel more alive than ever. I struck it lucky to have friends who recognised that, friends who knew when to start a kitchen disco.

One day, which felt like all other days, probably involving another episode of *Bargain Hunt*, I decided I should perhaps funnel my yawning expanse of time and frustration into something creative. My aunty, who had extended her stay with us after my diagnosis so she could fill my belly with yummy nutritious food, was a keen knitter, and as I watched her finish off yet another scarf or cardigan, I asked if she'd teach me to make something. Both she and Mum were over the moon to be able to fill my time and take my mind off everything cancer-related. When noticing my new-found hobby, other friends would send me wool and books with excellent titles such as *Stitch 'n Bitch*, happy to know they'd finally found a way to help me.

Suddenly I had a pretty intricate scarf-knitting project on the go. It was weirdly satisfying to have a project at all, and one that seemed achievable, if at times really frustrating. The rhythm of each stitch, the concentration each completed new row required, became meditative and enthralling and mind-numbing enough to sidetrack me from all the far greater stuff happening around me and to me. It was purple, green and blue and, yup, I was bloody chuffed when I finished it. I was glad to have seen a project through, a sense of achievement I hadn't actually felt in a while. But it didn't satisfy me completely. There was something niggling me that at first I couldn't put my finger on.

I started doing endless reading online about cancer patients in the same boat as me, scouring the internet for stories of people who lived a long time despite a 'terminal' diagnosis, fishing for those outliers. For me the stories where people had lived another twenty years became my benchmark – although ten would be great: *Just imagine the party we'd have for my cancerversary*, I thought. I know some people would have been happy with five, six . . . maybe I was greedy. I just knew that if it could be done, I would have something really tangible to hold on to. I needed proof that it was possible to live with cancer for a long time.

In my searches I came across blog after blog of personal experiences. I couldn't help but think how helpful a blog could be to update everyone on my health status. Instead of having to repeat myself over and over, I could simply write what was happening, from medical appointments to test results, so that when I did catch up with friends we could talk about anything *but* the cancer. So kriskancer.squarespace.com was born. Excuse me while I cringe, thinking about the way I wrote about my early cancer life – trust me, if those early words had been any use I would have just published the blog and not bothered with this book-writing lark. I spoke about cancer in a way I don't dare to now – you can sense my anger and sadness that I have since turned into more meaningful respect. The years have taught me that, and I can forgive the early-cancer Kris who didn't know better, or see things clearer.

Regardless, it achieved what I'd set out to achieve. My friends could follow my progress from afar and at the same time I was able to air thoughts and feelings, which felt like a good release. It gave me the chance to set the tone for how I would handle my treatment and uncertain future. And it ensured people resisted the well-meant urge to suggest I would recover because, trust me, what you don't want to hear after a terminal diagnosis is 'get well soon'.

The more I read, and the more complete strangers responded to my words in the blog, the more I felt something bigger brewing. One day I phoned a woman called Stefanie LaRue in America, as she'd told her secondary diagnosis story powerfully and successfully, and I wanted to see if she had any advice for me. I was nervous to quiz her, but I too wanted to share my story in a helpful way and I didn't have a clue how. Halfway through our conversation I remember her saying, 'Wait, you're calling me from the UK?' It didn't seem a big deal to me to be calling her from the other side of the world when, ya know, an email would have sufficed/been more normal since *who uses the phone these days*? And, thinking back, it probably was kinda intense. But I was suddenly so fixated on creating something that could help others – maybe, potentially, I mean, *who knows?* – *perhaps* not end up in the same sticky spot as me: a place where they are not told their cancer can't be cured because it was found too late. Whoa. There it was.

This nameless thing felt so overwhelmingly GINOR-MOUS but also like absolutely nothing, as I had no clue how I would make it a reality. I was just little ol' me. Little ol' Kris stuck at her mum's, jobless, with a body that was fighting the biggest fight of its life. Yet along with that sad reality another gallantly came forth: I had absolutely *nothing* to lose. Is it weird to admit that cancer came into my life when I had no loss to mourn? It was strangely liberating and freeing to have already experienced some of the worst things that can happen to you at the age of twenty-three. It created a fearlessness that made me almost untouchable. I allowed myself this thought: *Perhaps survival means more than not dying.*

Another day I was on a call to a lady called Wendy Watson, the first woman in the UK to have a preventive mastectomy, as she was a carrier of the faulty breast cancer gene – you know the one that was made famous after Angelina Jolie spoke openly about having it. Wendy's daughter Becky had been the youngest woman in the UK to have the op – essentially their entire family had been plagued with breast cancer and, being the feisty women they were, fought for preventive measures while also setting up the UK's first hereditary breast cancer helpline. Whatever it took for them to share their story and make change, I wanted a slice of it. What it took was encouragement. Wendy only had to tell me that I should, without a doubt, start something that didn't currently exist – a campaign that educated young people about breast cancer and the need to know their boobs – for me to think, *HOLY CRAP, maybe I should.*

*

Interesting fact: Maren and I were also throwing around ideas of a Meals on Wheels service at this time. Following a fun four weeks recreating our own version of *Come Dine With Me* (in which Maren made nettle soup and I triumphed with a winning Japanese meal) with our friends Jamie and Rach, we gained some inspiration and insight into the world of cancer-fighting foods: stuff that aids your body when it needs it most. Food you might not necessarily crave (hello chips and ice cream and salty things) but would defo keep your cells happy and ready for an onslaught of cancer drugs. My research had taken me down a lot of healthy-eating and cancer rabbit holes, and it pained me to think that patients weren't getting the information they needed, or any access to nutritious food that would boost their immune systems. All I ever got offered at the hospital was white-bread sandwiches, cakes or biscuits – great for comfort, not so good for giving your body the best possible chance to survive. We thought we could deliver meals to patients who needed them at the most critical time, during chemo, when they couldn't be arsed to cook, couldn't afford it, didn't have the energy to or didn't have the same support I did. Our early childhood playtimes working in our restaurant 'Maki' could have become an actual reality.

But that idea swiftly got swallowed up by another, and then another. In between popping pills to avoid chemo-induced nausea and painkillers to soothe my back pain –

which, post-radiotherapy, had improved a lot – I was making phone call after phone call, writing email after email. I was possessed by an almost manic (possibly fuelled by the steroids), crazy energy – but better crazy than dead, I thought. Any cancer charity that allowed me to share my story through an online form received a sermon on my life thus far. The more positive feedback I received to an idea that wasn't even an idea yet, the more my hunger for something big and transformative grew.

Two weeks after my first of eight chemotherapy sessions, I was sitting at my mum's dining table with seven of my friends, plus Maren, Mum and Maike, and one pal on Skype, as she'd contracted a cold and was therefore banned from the meeting in case my now immuno-suppressed body caught it. We didn't have enough chairs for everyone, but we huddled together both physically and mentally. Here was a group of people who, without knowing it, were helping me more than any ball of wool or body lotion could. They were helping me birth an idea that was burning my insides, my purpose bubbling beneath, yelling a bid for life.

Of course there was silliness, of course we drew boobs on a piece of paper, of course I made light of a seemingly terrifying situation to ease the mood (I was really tremen-dously good at that), but we also talked about ways in which we could start a campaign that might just encourage people – our people, all our friends and people of our age – to check their boobs.

'Cop a feel. What do you think about that for a name?' I asked sheepishly, knowing its connotations to unsolicited groping.

'Great.'

'Brilliant.'

'Spot on.'

These were not the responses I was expecting. It wasn't until perhaps a few months later that I discovered the unspoken power that comes with having cancer. People are far too afraid to upset you, and this may well have been one of those occasions. I would harness that power, I noted.

'We could turn what some might think of as a bit of a risqué, inappropriate turn of phrase into something that makes people actually check their boobs, like hijacking it and giving it a whole new meaning. A life-saving meaning.' Again, no one disagreed. 'That's settled then. Oh – and I think we should spell it with a K.'

For some reason I had become obsessed with spelling cancer with a K. My name was spelled with a K, yet so often it was misspelled with a C. I'd already shortened it to Kris because it saved my energy. I wanted to give cancer that same level of annoyance I had felt. Why should it get to be spelled correctly when my name wasn't? Was I cute or a knob? Luckily someone did have the balls to argue against this idea. Cop a Feel, after a few more Facebook messages back and forth, later became CoppaFeel!, not because any branding professionals advised us towards that decision, but simply, well, because we thought it sounded and looked better. And it was spelt with a C.

No one at that table that day in May 2009 had the foggiest about how to start an awareness campaign. No one had useful contacts. My friend Adam had set up his own website for selling stoves and wood burners, so knew how to get our site 'hosted', whatever that meant. Ben was at law school. Rach was in the early stages of becoming a doctor. Jamie was at the start of a budding marketing career. Lou worked for the local council. The others were friends who believed in me. You will never find that combination of people in any manual on how to start a charity, but I can tell you that no experience or knowledge is as powerful as simply having belief in making the seemingly impossible possible.

If you are reading this and recognising some familiar niggles – a similar burning need to change something, to raise hell about some injustice, or feel the need to add your voice to 'cancer awareness' – I need you to stop for a minute. Very often I get asked how to start a campaign or charity: someone will want to replicate what I have done to make a positive change in their arena – whether that's ovarian cancer or mental health. I ask you to do this thing for me: *take a deep breath*. There's no need to jump into anything right now. Yes, that fire is *lit*, but use that heat wisely. I gave myself *no* time to grieve the loss of the former me. I gave myself no time to simply 'be'. I've learned that now, eleven years on, and I've been granted an opportunity to do everything I might have done then, now. I have been granted time to *live*. What if all you do is get angry, do some campaigning and miss the chance to breathe in life?

Also, let's not waste your time or other people's time or money. If you see a glaring big gap in the market for a campaign, that's one thing, but if someone else is already fighting the fight you want to fight, then ask them how you can join in. Are they doing it badly? Could they be doing it better? Have you got some *amazing* ideas for how to do it more effectively? Great. Ask to have a chat. I learned early on as a charity boss to accept advice and guidance because, believe it or not, I didn't always know best or get it right. I didn't always have solutions; I couldn't always see things from the perspective it needed to be seen from. Offer your brilliant mind and thoughts to others: it may be more valuable than you think. Surviving cancer isn't about running a marathon, or 'wearing it pink', or starting a charity! It's about knowing how to 'be', without feeling a constant need to 'do'.

Don't yield to that pressure and just allow time for healing. I'm a sucker for a good Instagram quote and I read one the other day by astrologer and writer Chani Nicholas which sums this up pretty well: 'You don't have to heal yourself into a neat little story of triumph or success. Life is messy. Growth isn't linear. You are not a commercial.'

You'll soon discover, or may already have some inkling, that my need to start CoppaFeel! stretched *way* beyond saving lives and ensuring that what happened to me didn't happen to others. It was needed – OH HECK, it was needed – but I needed it every bit as much as you, the world, did. I didn't see this at the time, but I see that clearly now.

I've digressed. Let's get back to it.

Maren and her uni pal Hugo were staying at Mum's, working remotely for Cornwall Council on various landscaping projects. Both were exceptional garden designers following their first-class degrees, with bright, award-winning futures ahead of them (so much so they would go on to design a CoppaFeel! show garden at the prestigious Hampton Court Palace Flower Show in 2011 and win gold! Hugo Bugg is now a pretty big name in the garden-design world and let me take this moment to gush about HOW PROUD I AM OF HIM). I was glad to have them home, as I needed to voice the ideas whirling through my head and also because it was their company that I craved during moments when, occasionally, I remembered I had cancer.

While they were with me, they got to work on our logo as well as a website. Once we had a few designs whittled down, we printed them off to show the world. By 'the world' I obviously mean anyone we harangued into talking to us in Daventry town centre, outside Waitrose, Costa Coffee and Savers, to be precise. We asked them how the designs made them feel, whether they were relevant for a campaign asking you to check your boobs, and any other feedback, good or bad. We were desperate for any and all words they had to offer. I look back and wonder where I found the guts to do this. Where I found the ballsy confidence to shove logo designs in front of unsuspecting strangers to get the answers I needed to help move this thing forward.

Not long after our highly professional tactical marketing research, we settled on the most popular design: the design that still exists today, albeit much more defined and professional-looking (no offence, Hugo and Mar!).

Next we needed to somehow get our message out to young people. Sharing it on Facebook wasn't enough; we needed to be face to face, up close and personal with them. 'Them' being these innocent earthlings who didn't yet have a clue that checking their boobs could save their life. Spring was sprinting into summer and with it came our long-planned visit to Beach Break Live Festival in Port Lympne in Kent (yeah, weird name for a landlocked location. It's a long story but, fine, since you asked: their previous beachside home in Cornwall didn't want them back). What better place than a student-only festival to speak to young folk about boobs? It would be the ultimate test: if we could get through to fun-searching, post-exam-stressed, desperate-to-let-off-steam-and-drink-and-shag students, then surely we'd be on to a winner. The only hurdle would be actually getting a pitch at said festival without money, without any experience of carrying out what I guess you could call 'health-awareness activation' (one chat with a marketeer and I became a marketing wanker) or contacts. What we lacked in experience and physical means, we made up for in sublime naivety and persuasive email writing.

A swift response from the Beach Break team said a very baffling YES. We had got ourselves a pitch, at a festival, to talk to people about boobs. We laughed for a moment before realising we also did not have any promo materials, or structure to house such promotional materials. Not so much as a table.

Jamie, my good friend from school and aforementioned marketing friend, had a plan. But first I have to tell you how fundamental he was in the success of the charity. He would be the one to create our entire brand, hone our 'personality' and sail us through some of the roughest storms, and today he is the chair of trustees for CoppaFeel! I don't know if he really knew what he was letting himself in for when he casually offered to help me, but his commitment has been unwavering. A.K.A. he is amazing. So Jamie, on a mission, decided it would be absolutely plausible to waltz in to Homebase, ask for the manager, explain our situation and receive a gazebo completely free of charge. I'm sure you can guess that this did not happen. It became a standing joke, a warm memory, and in fact the word 'gazebo' was several passwords to CoppaFeel! accounts (that have since changed, before you rush to hack us and bleed us dry).

My friend Niall, the same Niall who drove to see me from Scotland the day after my diagnosis, donated a van, a perfect white Ford Transit Connect that would become our vehicle to carry out awareness work, but more than that, it became freedom and independence on wheels for me. That van helped me metaphorically feel a little less stuck in mud until, of course, we did get it physically stuck in mud one very wet day at another festival later that summer.

Jamie and I were the first to arrive on site the day before Beach Break officially started. As we sat in the midday sun cutting out stickers of our logo from huge rolls, several site staff popped by and asked what we were up to. I guess it might have looked a little strange, this girl with no hair perched on the floor cutting out stickers while everyone else was erecting their elaborate food, drink or shop stalls. Sandwiched in the middle of it was our little (paid for) gazebo, which we magically got printed up with our design just in time. We had T-shirts too, T-shirts with our logo on, thanks to Jamie's cousins. We couldn't have felt more unofficially official.

Our entourage followed soon after, made up of Maren, Hugo and some of their university mates. All boys. All handsome, which we thought could work in our favour when getting girls (or boys) to come to our little stall to speak to us. That's about as thought-out as we had got. We had focused so much energy and excitement on actually getting there, with T-shirts, wo-man power and some posters (stuck to some display material we'd borrowed from Maren's boyfriend Graham, who was, conveniently, a pharmaceutical rep), that we'd forgotten to plan out what we would say to people, and how we would broach the subject of boobs with complete strangers.

The festival floodgates opened on a beautiful, bright sunny day. Wearing our T-shirts, we looked like we were such a team, a force for potential good. As people came by to ask what we were doing, we'd start talking about CoppaFeel! as if we'd been around for a while, as if we actually knew what we were doing. Of course we were nervous at first, but it wasn't long before we morphed into people who sounded like they knew what they were talking about. We may have faked our professionalism, but one thing was real: my cancer diagnosis. I was there, with secondary breast cancer, something that could have been avoided had I maybe checked my boobs. Using me as the hook helped make people understand it all much better. They'd leave with one of our freshly cut handprint stickers affixed to their boob to carry on the rest of their carefree festival experience.

Nothing we said could have, or should have, scared them. We weren't giving medical advice – anyone who believed they had a symptom of breast cancer was swiftly told to see their GP when they got home. We were there to empower. We improvised something that now sounds so creepy: 'Dr Cop' sessions, which involved Jamie wearing a doctor's white coat demonstrating how to check on our friend Louis's chest. We'd painted a fake six-pack on his abs and he donned a pink wig to complete the look.

This was Maren's and my third year at Beach Break Live and each time we travelled with face paints (these were the days before glitter, guys!). We would paint pretty flowery designs or abstract shapes on our faces. Finding a use for them to make out that Louis had a way more toned bod (his stipulation) was one thing, but shortly after that came another use, when a passer-by spotted our masterpieces in progress. 'How much for face paint?' they asked, assuming we were a face-painting set-up. Baffled but simultaneously spotting an opportunity, we replied: 'Donation. Give what you like.' And there, ladies and gents, is how we started fundraising for CoppaFeel!. That is where we made our very first pennies.

We were not a charity at this point, but the idea to become one had crossed our minds. The word *charity* didn't sit right with me back then. To me charity felt so stuffy, so stagnant, and that's not what I wanted Coppa-Feel! to be. I wanted us to solve a problem, get in and get out. I always wanted there to be a sense of urgency, a feeling that we'd get the job done. Of course, I didn't know then how useful being a charity could be, and that we'd need to consider it in order to operate legally and credibly. So although we hadn't discussed it at great length, we did know that in order to become one, we had to secure £5,000 from who knows where. Our tiny, crappy gazebo suddenly became a hive of face and body (on request) painting.

Lucky for the recipients, most of our gang were design-ers and had *some* training, if not of the face-painting variety. Miraculously no one complained, everyone donated and, most importantly of all, everyone listened because, well, they couldn't get away once they'd commit-ted to having their face turned into a piece of art. It gave us five to ten minutes, depending on who was painting (some of the paintings were so extensive the poor bugger could have been diagnosed with breast cancer and recov-ered in that time). During those minutes we'd ask them whether they'd ever thought about checking their boobs.

It led to healthy conversations that in turn, we hoped, led to a whole new behaviour and attitude change. I, with a bald and colourfully painted bonce, was proof that it happens. Getting breast cancer at a young age was no longer something they might one day read about in a magazine or one of those annoying Facebook clickbait stories, but right in front of them with a tiger face.

I came alive. Every conversation I had or saw my friends having made my insides explode. I couldn't help but consider that maybe, perhaps, *who knows*, but *potentially* someone would head home from the festival and check their boobs – bloody hell, they might even have a fondle with themselves in their tents that very evening. Every penny someone popped in our scrappy little red bucket, which I'd pleaded with my friend to bring along even though we had not expected to fundraise, I felt myself grow into someone I did not recognise: someone who had, perhaps, maybe, *who knows*, but *potentially* found a purpose. I was scared to think this, but I thought it anyway.

The word of our little face-painting, boob-checking venture spread. Without our knowledge, the site staff were asking all VIP guestlist attendees entering the festival to donate money to CoppaFeel! at the gates. They told all artists performing that we, this little tiny gazebo, a girl with no hair and her pals, were on a mission to save lives. I'd love to know what exactly they said to them, but whatever it was somehow convinced festival headliners the Zutons to dedicate 'Valerie' to me. There we were, standing in the crowd, ready to shake off and let loose after a long day talking and painting in the sun, when we heard the words: 'There's a girl in the audience called Kris. This song is for her.' I leapt ten feet in the air. My friends all stared at me, Maren burst out laughing, and I probably went bright red. A song. Dedicated to me. ME.

I'd never felt such conflicting emotions – I felt so happy to be held in such regard to get a stage shout-out, such joy to be among this congregation of dancing strangers who knew about a girl called Kris, but simultaneously wanted the ground to swallow me up there and then and quickly. The guitar strumming started pumping up through my feet, now in time with my own heartbeat. I was scooped up onto the shoulders of our tallest friend, James. There was such palpable joy in the air. It was so organic, and throbbed with life like I'd never experienced it before, a million light years away from the torment of cancer or heartache.

It didn't stop there. The following day the Cuban Brothers would tell the crowd to check their boobs, and that same evening Maren and I found ourselves in the dressing room of Dizzee Rascal. That sounds more rock and roll than it was. We bumbled our way through, explaining what we were doing there and why people should check their boobs, to which he replied: 'You're beautiful.' I was too shy to respond with anything other than thanks. I was so confused. I couldn't really compute what was happening but, man, I loved it. I was experiencing a buzz and joy that I just wasn't familiar with. It all felt so new. The main-stage MC and host even found me in the crowd to say: 'I've read about people like you, but I've never met them, until now.'

That sentence, and the sincerity all over his face, has never left me. It was all I could think about for the rest of our time there, all I could think about as my heart raced from all the adrenaline when I was trying to sleep (in the back of the van) and all I could think about on the way home. Well, that's a lie: I'd also met a v. cute boy who was occupying many thoughts too, but more on that later. What had the MC meant? Was my story really that extraordinary? I half believed it was – why else would I have gone to all this effort to share it with so many in a field in Kent? But his comment had made me look at myself and my value and my worth like I had never done before. His words danced around in my head. He might have been off his face and not recall ever speaking to me or even meeting me, but regardless, he handed me permission to be liked, to be admired, to be looked up to. Maybe that's a knobbish thing to say (it certainly felt knobbish to write), but his words helped release something in me that had until then felt so very hidden, almost forbidden, so tight and locked away.

As I floated around the site, people were giving me strange looks and I began to think that this buzz I was experiencing was oozing out of me and was really obvious to others, almost like my body had become a loudhailer shouting: MAKE WAY! THIS GIRL IS ALIIIIVE FOR THE FIRST TIME EVER!! In retrospect they were probably just looking at my shiny bald noggin. I wasn't drinking because I'd heard cancer drugs and alcohol don't mix too well, but even if I could have had alcohol, I didn't feel any need to. I was, wait for it: drunk on life.

It gets more nauseating: on a Ferris-wheel ride with Maren I remember closing my eyes and letting the warm air hit my face. I wanted to absorb all the feelings and bathe in every single one. I felt I was seeing life in a whole new way. Each spin of the wheel supercharging my energy, recharging the vigour I had expended on every-thing and everyone but myself for so long, filling up a sort of reserve, a bucket of power I didn't know existed. Some new, unfamiliar feeling really struck me: I felt complete. Weird, given that I was recently told my body was falling to pieces. Somehow it was enough to convince me that I would be OK, that it was already more than OK. Every spin of the wheel was drawing a line under the life that had preceded that moment; life burst into every bit of me that I had shut down pre-cancer. Once you are faced with the fact that death is a real thing, there's not really much else left to fear, is there? And, knowing that, who would ever dare to have power over me again? As the ever-so-great author of *The Cancer Journals* Audre Lorde, once wrote in the seventies: 'If the life spark kept burning there would be fuel.'

There was something very mighty about being so high above the festival, above the world, above the shitshow of cancer. It allowed a perspective shift that I didn't know I needed. I stepped off that Ferris wheel a new woman, a woman who started to question whether it was living with cancer for many years that she wanted or whether it was the LIFE in those years she should be striving for. And fuck, did I like her.

I only really came back down to earth physically and metaphorically when I had to pull down my trousers in the back of the van and stick a needle in my leg to inject myself with something called GCSF, a little boost to help my bloods and thus my immune system stay happy ahead of my next chemotherapy dose. (A festival site isn't the most sanitary place for someone with a compromised immune system, but hand sanitiser became, and still is, my BFF.)

That dreaded manky Monday morning of the end of the festival dawned and it was time to pack up. Nothing about the end of that weekend was sad, though. It was *so* far from an ending – I mean, something absurd had just begun. We headed to the site crew for final goodbyes. We'd become so close with two site staff legends named Ofir and Lulu that they felt like family. It was only then that they revealed all the fundraising they'd been doing behind the scenes and handed over a box full of cash. A box with £700 in it. The most money I had ever seen in one go. I think I wept. I think I said thank you over and over again. I think I smiled so much my face hurt. I think I realised what pride and love and gratitude all mashed together felt like. We left the festival smellier, sunburnt, happier and more determined than ever before.

The Cancer Poster Girl

*So I said I'd keep you updated and that I shall do!
I had my final lot of EC chemo drugs (epirubicin
and cyclophosphamide) on Wednesday. I'm pretty
happy to see the back of that stuff! Although in
three weeks' time I'll be on the harder stuff, which
they'll be pumping into me every two weeks, which
is nasty, as this gives my body less time to recover
for the next onslaught. However, that just means I'll
get this buggering treatment out of the way quicker.
I'm having daily injections again to ensure my
blood count stays nice and happy. Mar was taught
how to inject me today, which was possibly more
scary for her than me ... I'm feeling my usual
drugged-up not-myself, which is commonly associ-
ated with chemo. Nothing I can't handle, though.
And my bastard breasticle tumour has shrunk*

another 1 cm *does tumour shrinkage dance* Soooo folks, you are officially updated on kristin's kancerthon . . .

Back home we gathered our thoughts as much as we could. It took me a while to come down from the high of Beach Break. I replayed the song shout-outs and just about every conversation in my head, my thoughts whirling like a washing machine. I couldn't wait to get back out there and keep this elation alive. But first I needed more rounds of chemo.

And, in between, Jamie and I decided it was time to get some real education on breast awareness. Sure, what we'd read online was legit enough to get us through chats we were having in festival fields, but we really wanted to get to grips with what one of the major breast cancer charities in the UK was advocating for people older than me. Breast Cancer Care had developed a course called 'Train the Trainer', in which medical professionals like nurses could get the lowdown on all things breast health. The course wasn't necessarily for complete novices who didn't already work in the field, and probably not for someone recently diagnosed with breast cancer and her pal, but we were welcomed nonetheless. They were pleased to finally have the first bloke in attendance too. We learned everything from how breast cancer risk factors are portrayed in the media to the anatomy of the breast. In particular I learned how much I hated the term 'breasts'. I much prefer 'boobs'. Although they couldn't help us with *how* we would get this stuff across to people our age, the course leaders were keen to hear of our festival escapades and heady future plans.

We applied for more festivals that summer and found ourselves in more fields, with more friends, painting more faces, and having more conversations about boobs. As our activities ramped up, so did the effect the chemotherapy was having on my body. The drug concoction I was given can impact every patient very differently. The myriad common side effects were handy to know about, but were by no means exhaustive or true to reality. I'd somehow manage to time my outings at festivals with 'good weeks'. I'd get a dose, lie low for a week and, just as I was coming out the other side, I'd have enough energy to put cancer aside for a weekend before starting it all again. As time went on, chemotherapy had a cumulative effect, and the good weeks shortened into the odd good day here and there.

It was when we were at Farmfest that I noticed how much things had shifted. I spent most of my time horizontal in the back of the van, back doors wide open so I could see all my worker bees churning out facial masterpieces, and having boob chat after boob chat. I must have been a sorry sight. Here was a group of people trying to empower people about their health when I looked anything but healthy. I was worried that my pale and now dry and scaly skin (thanks to the chemo) and the dark circles around my eyes would scare people rather than make them feel proactive about their boob health. Maren would bring me a plate of delights that usually consisted of avocados, smoked mackerel and maybe some sweetcorn, washed down with some juice with wheatgrass powder mixed in – we spared no trouble or expense to ensure I consumed proper nutrients. I conserved my strength, injected myself with GCSF and napped. As evening came I'd stored up enough energy to crawl out of my hovel to try and enjoy the festival. I wanted so badly to be like everyone else: care- and pain-free.

With my energy taking a nosedive and fatigue making an unwelcome entrance, we decided to keep our awareness-raising efforts closer to home. Friends would hold bake sales at work that would help get us ever closer to our £5k target for opening a charity. We had by this point sent off our application to the Charity Commission. Our mission was now clear and our objectives sounded punchy, scarily grown-up but absolutely achievable. We threw together a trustee board made up of me, Maren, Jamie and Rach, while Mum became the company secretary. So sure were we that we could create something brilliant, our naivety and all-out blag never once slowed our efforts or enthusiasm. A fact I learned along the way is that without naivety you'd never try.

One day I got a call from a patient-advocate person at Cancer Research UK (CRUK). I had totally forgotten that during my early stages of research I'd submitted my story into any and every website form that I could in the hope someone would reply and, I dunno, maybe validate that my story was worth sharing. Maybe hearing it from my biased family and friends wasn't enough for me. They were calling about a new TV advert they were working on and wondered if I might be keen to feature. Obviously I was. I played it cool, though: 'I'll have to check my diary.' WHO had I become!?

I'd already done some filming. Just after my first round of chemo, presenter and writer Dawn O'Porter had made a documentary about hereditary breast cancer. We'd filmed at my house and even at hospital, during a long and arduous chemo appointment. I was no savvy media queen, but the camera and interview questions didn't challenge me in the slightest. I had absolutely nothing to hide; hiding had got me into this mess.

CRUK called to fill me in on the advert filming, and an email followed containing the script. I was prepared for it to be hard-hitting – anything I'd ever seen on telly about cancer was. The fact I'd been chosen to give the last and most impactful punch-you-in-the-nuts line at first escaped me. It wasn't until I was sitting in a very fancy location house in West London saying the words: 'Because as yet, it isn't a fight we always win,' into a camera lens that was unnervingly close to my face that I realised the impact of those words. I was young, I had no hair: I represented the true tragedy of a cancer diagnosis. I was the poster girl for it.

I didn't mind; of course I didn't. I would have done anything to help make someone act on any cancer symptoms, stop anyone from being in my shoes and also give money to cancer research. At that point I had no boundaries. Their approach was a formula that I guess worked: hit the public hard, make them donate. But inside I wasn't the girl they were portraying on a TV advert.

Featuring in the advert also connected me with my first ever fellow younger breast cancer patient, called Erica, who would become my late-night chemo-side-effect freak-out outlet. She was a calming and reassuring voice of reason because she had already been through the same treatment. It was only later when I finally got to meet her, at the Maggie's Centre in London, that I realised that not only was she a bloody brilliant confidante in my hour of need but a beyond vivacious and hilarious one too. I feel lucky to say that we're still friends today.

I was learning the 'share my story with anyone who'd listen' trade. I soon befriended the PR person at CRUK, called Jane. She put me forward for article after article off the back of the advert.

So one day, when Jane asked me whether I'd let them film me at home for a case-study story, I thought little of it. It just seemed like a nice and important thing to do. By this point the chemo was starting to hit me harder. Days became more of a blur and I struggled with motivation. The morning the crew were due to arrive at my house, Maren scanned the outfit choice I'd made and asked me if I was planning to get changed for the filming. I wasn't. I was also puzzled by the suggestion. What was wrong with my garms? She shrugged. She, Maike and Mum had gone to a weirdly big effort, though. Mum even wore make-up.

On this particular day I almost couldn't be bothered. It was a struggle to muster any enthusiasm; my face was so crusty it hurt to smile. The chemo was draining me. I looked tired, I felt tired and I was struggling to see the end of it all. I'd find myself asking how long this was actually going to go on for. I had a finish line for chemo: 5 August 2009. We had a rough timescale between finishing chemo and allowing my body to recover before having my boob removed. We didn't know yet if I might need radiotherapy straight after to zap up any remaining cancer cells in my chest, but it was likely. And then what? Who could say whether these five months of chemo were enough to keep cancer quiet for a while? The weight of these internal questions and dilemmas, coupled with drugs and fatigue, dragged me down mentally and physically. It was no surprise that I cared so little about my outfit choice that day. Plus, why would it matter what I wore when I was told the video was to be used for some internal case-study work? But I did feel ugly and no outfit change would help with that. It didn't help that Maren had just got back from a long, dreamy trip tandem cycling with Graham around the Alps. We'd never looked so different, so not like twins. She was bronzed and lean, I was a bloated blob and ghostlike. Ugh.

A tiny, energetic and funny woman called Nicola was producing the video along with tall, dark-haired Yvonne. Then with them they brought a crew and Jane was there for support. It seemed a bit much for something so small fry. It was a beautiful summer day, so we conducted Mum, Maike and Maren's interviews in the garden. I stayed inside waiting and once it was my turn we chose my bedroom for my interview. They asked me everything about my diagnosis, how it all felt, if I was proud of my achievements thus far. I thought that was it but then was told a photographer was arriving shortly to take photos too. Again, I was surprised at the lengths they were going to, but also not surprised enough to question it. I didn't quite have enough energy and interest to poke them for more information, I just told myself it was important to be able to keep sharing my story. *The more people that hear it, the more lives we save*, is all I thought for most of that year, and it became my way to cope.

'We want to showcase more of your work with Coppa-Feel! We want to see you in action, for this case-study film,' they told me. A whole day's worth of filming was, bizarrely, not enough. We didn't have any more festivals lined up – well, at least not for the time frame in which they wanted to get this shot. I was disappointed not to be able to show them some real interactions like the ones we were having in festival fields, but suggested that maybe they could film us having a meeting. A catch-up meeting with the same friends who had been helping me until now.

Fast-forward a week or so and we find ourselves at The Hoxton hotel in East London. A far, far cry from my mum's living room. It was so plush, so London, so everything our little grassroots campaign was not – yet. They'd arranged everything. I wanted it to be as useful and real as possible despite the fact they wouldn't actually be capturing much of what I was saying, more what I was doing: looking serious, talking updates, strategy, plans ahead, a girl completely blagging it. A girl with cancer getting the hell on with her mission to save lives, never really knowing if what she was doing was having any impact whatsoever. I saw it as an opportunity to hold an actual meeting and update friends on stuff we'd been doing since I last spoke to them and what I needed help with next. We chatted about universities, festival ideas, fundraising ideas, our impending half-marathon, a dance-a-thon event happening in Cornwall, how I'd just managed to score £1,000 from a local Avon Foundation fund – an organisation that supports women to lead safe and healthy lives – to put towards our ever-growing charity pot. I took it all really seriously; it's as if I had to prove to the cameras that I was, like, a real campaign director.

'Kristin, Kristin, is that you?' came a deranged voice shouting from the entrance of the hotel. I looked over, and in pant-shitting horror realised it was Andy and Lou from *Little Britain*. In full costume. Heading straight towards me. And they were still saying my name.

'Kristin, you have won a Pride of Britain award – congratulations!' 'Lou', a.k.a. David Walliams, said.

'I've what?'

I looked around and my friends and family were by this point all grinning and smiling and cheering, while I was sitting frozen to the sofa. I could not compute what was happening. The cameras were rolling, capturing every bit of my reaction. They handed me an envelope with my invite to the awards night.

The rest is quite a blur. I remember Andy and Lou breaking out of character eventually once the cameras were off and telling me how brilliant they thought my work with CoppaFeel! was. They were so kind, so complimentary, and I was still so confused. Who had schemed this? It was revealed to me that Jane from CRUK, Nicola and Yvonne (who were not from CRUK but in fact producers from ITV), Mum, Maike and Maren were all in on it. They'd been told weeks ago and were sworn to secrecy. The day they did the filming for that 'internal case study' stuff was a recording for the actual awards night, to be televised on ITV. I'd been well and truly tricked. I was also well and truly FUMING that Mar hadn't forced me into better clothes or even *some* make-up that day they came to our house. The effort my family had gone to to make themselves look nice for the TV broadcast suddenly made so much sense.

Mum couldn't wait to admit that she'd been desperate to tell me I'd won, but didn't want to spoil the surprise. So much effort had gone into that very moment, she couldn't bear to let the producers down. But she had also really struggled watching me hit a wall with chemotherapy. There were days where I'd only leave my bed to go to the loo, and even that felt like climbing a mountain. The drugs pumped relentlessly through my system, killing every good and bad cell in their path. Those groundhog days, when there was no sign of me getting any more alive than the day before, were when she had *almost* burst out that I'd won a Pride of Britain award just to lift my spirits. She'd have done anything for that. But she hadn't, and I'm so relieved because, despite my A for

GCSE drama, acting surprised for TV would have been *awkward* at best, untelevisable at worst.

The awards were just around the corner and so planning my outfit became my new distraction. We arranged a shopping trip at the Bullring in Birmingham, where I tried on countless outfits before settling on a strapless number from Monsoon with green suede strappy shoes and a matching clutch bag. I'd already decided I wouldn't be wearing my wig. As I neared the end of chemo my hair was already starting to come back. Little wispy chick-like hair was beginning to sprout; I remember I first noticed it when a gust of wind hit it and I was startled by the sensation of wind in my hair. Maren and I decided I'd need a spray tan because I looked practically dead. My skin had become so sensitive to everything that I'd shielded myself from the sun all summer for fear of burning to a crisp. Some days I walked around with my face covered in sexy Sudocrem.

The thing about spray tans is that you have to wait for them to develop, and you can't wash the initial streaky tan off too soon or you will just remove it entirely. It wasn't my first spray tan rodeo, but this time for some reason I had especially obvious patches all over me. People who are not me would likely not make plans following a spray tan until it looks natural.

But I am me, and unfortunately my very first Coppa-Feel! talk, which Jamie and I had planned for weeks, fell on one of the most tan-developing days of all. There we were, standing in my old school, of all places, presenting to students who were sitting exactly where I had just a few years before. I hoped they'd be more distracted by my bald head or my commitment to the denim miniskirt, tights and cowboy-boot combo I still hadn't moved on from.

In all seriousness, though, that moment was a biggie. I couldn't help but think of the impact we might be having on the girl sitting where I once sat. The girl who was learning something that might change the way she thinks about her boobs. Might help her feel OK about talking about them, touching them, noticing them if things seem odd. Perhaps she'd go on to speak about whatever she notices and stand up for her health. Maybe she would do everything that I didn't. Everything that would ensure she didn't have to stand in front of a group of young people with a bald, tan-lined head sharing a story about that time she should have checked her boobs. We couldn't tell from any of their faces if what we were saying would turn them into proactive little health heroes or if we scared them or bored them. But they were silent, and apparently that was a good thing.

To this day I still prefer speaking with adults, as I at least get some facial expressions and the odd chuckle out of them; kids not so much. We've obviously since perfected our school-talk delivery and know, from

THE CANCER POSTER GIRL

feedback, that it does sink in. We know that despite the silence and startled-rabbit faces they go off and talk about what they've just heard. I hoped and longed for those little corridor conversations among friends, discussing boobs like it was as commonplace as discussing what was in their sandwiches that day.

The awards wasn't just the ceremony. As winners, you get put up in a fancy hotel, you have a winners' dinner the night before, hosted by Carol Vorderman, you have the day of the awards to enjoy London, and then you get ready and hop on the winners' bus to the Grosvenor House Hotel on Park Lane. We'd planned the awards day to a tight schedule. I'd managed to squeeze in a massage at a place called Silver Pearl, owned by a wonder woman named Rachel who had set it up to allow people with cancer to have free holistic treatments paid for by clients who didn't have cancer. The salon was just off crazy-busy Bond Street, a safe haven tucked away and a moment to breathe and gather my thoughts ahead of a whirlwind evening. I played out scenes of tripping up as I walked to the stage, ugly crying as they announced my name, but most of all I just really wanted that moment to be worthwhile for CoppaFeel! and its future. After all, *a lot* more people were about to hear about it.

*

Back at the hotel we'd arranged for a lovely make-up artist to make me look less tired and frazzled. I'd met Lucy on a shoot Maren and I did for *Glamour* magazine. On that occasion she'd been instructed not to put any make-up on me other than foundation. No blusher, no nothing that made me look like I wasn't dying of cancer, while Maren was allowed to be as done up as she liked. I was put in a frumpy grey T-shirt while Mar was put in a dress. They were, you guessed it, emphasising my cancer-ness. The bald head was clearly not enough: they needed to ramp up the visual drama by making identical twins look anything but.

To this day it's the most depressing photo shoot I've ever done and if I'd had the balls I grew at some point later on, I would have told them to stick it. But I didn't. I was knackered from the chemo and had no fight in me, so I tried to remember the 'greater good'. I badly wanted false eyelashes, as mine had fallen out and I was crap at applying them myself. Lovely Lucy agreed to stick some on once the photos were taken; she hung around long enough so I could at least leave the shoot feeling a little better. We stayed in touch and I knew if anyone could make me look and feel at least half decent for the awards, it would be her.

I got to take Maren, Graham, Mum, Maike and Jamie as guests to the awards. What happened that evening deserves a whole chapter for itself, but I'm going to bullet point some key moments for you:

- Getting an unsolicited boob grope from Hannah Waterman, a.k.a. Laura Beale from *EastEnders*.
- Featherweight champion Barry McGuigan giving me a high-five.
- Meeting and falling in love with every member of dance troupe Diversity.
- Dannii Minogue telling Maren and I that our relationship reminded her of hers and Kylie's.
- Esther Rantzen being the only person I did not know but the only person Graham did.
- Des Lynam calling Mar the 'ugly twin'. LOL. Man, we still laugh so hard about this today.
- Louis Walsh calling Maren Diana Vickers.
- Getting stood up by Dermot O'Leary, who was supposed to be sitting next to me, only to then make him feel really bad about it and know he'd be an ambassador for CoppaFeel! one day.
- Crucially, I did not fall over. In fact, I was practically floating on the clapping and whooping (coming from my table), and the adrenaline, and Sigur Rós's 'Hoppípolla', which was playing.

All that is fun to read, isn't it? I'd got so caught up in the showbizzy glamour in the lead-up to the event and on the night that it only dawned on me how much of a fraud I actually was once I was on that stage. Perhaps it was the other stories of war veterans saving people from near death and lifetime achievements that included inventing the MRI machine that had me wondering what THE FUCK I was doing there. I hadn't yet proven *anything*. I'd started a blog; I'd shared my story; I was featured on a TV advert for CRUK; I went to a few festivals and told people to check their boobs. I am not being bashful. I had genuinely not shown you, and by 'you' I guess I mean the people who ultimately decided I should win this award, that I had made the impact I was planning and dreaming to make. I mean, how could I? It had been just eight months since I'd been told I had cancer! And having cancer, I need to say, is not honourable.

So yeah, I didn't feel deserving, but I did feel motivated. I still had *so* much to prove, so much to show the world about the difference boob chat or no boob chat can have on young people. So much to teach people about the consequence of a late diagnosis, so much to validate why I, Kris Hallenga, had got cancer in the first place. And I can't deny that being handed an award by Baby Spice and Scary Spice on prime-time TV helped.

Friends in High Places
(With Too Many Christmas Trees)

Just after finding out I'd won the award, I received this email:

Kris,

I hope you don't mind me contacting you out of the blue, but I've been reading about and hugely inspired by your work! I'm sure you are already exhausted at the thought of Breast Cancer Awareness Month looming, but I hope you don't mind me adding to your list of things to think about! We are going to have a reception here, on 8 October, to celebrate all the amazing things that people are doing at the moment to help beat breast cancer. We were wondering, firstly, if you would be free to join us, but also if there are, say, around ten others that you'd like us to invite who have been involved with your efforts in some way? Trustees, partners, volunteers, celebrity endorsers – whomever it would be most useful for you to be able to thank in this way. If that sounds like it could work for you, if you get me email addresses for them I can process them so they are issued with a formal e-invite. Would be fantastic if some of your supporters could join us.

Best wishes,
Kirsty

Kirsty McNeill
10 Downing St, SW1A 2AA

Did I mind a special adviser in Downing Street contacting me? About an invite to No. 10? I reread it several times, convinced it was a hoax. I forwarded it to Jamie and Maren and giggled with hysteria. Not only was I going to be on telly, but in the same week I was going to be taking ten mates to No. 10. I later learned that when you win a Pride of Britain award you actually get to go to No. 10 the morning after as well. So I found myself at said famous address twice within the space of two weeks.

Once I'd replied to Kirsty with a nonchalant 'I guess I could be free', I received my official invite:

25 September 2009

Dear Kristan

The Prime Minister and Sarah Brown would like to invite you to a reception at Downing Street, to celebrate Breast Cancer Awareness Month and the progress made in beating breast cancer, on Thursday 8 October 2009, 6.00 p.m.–8.00 pm.
    Could you please reply to this email with the best postal address for us to send your official invitation card to.

Thank you,
Rosemarie Brim
Events & Visits Office
10 Downing Street

In fact it was Rosemarie (who misspelled my name, but I will let that slide) who, at the reception, would mention how nice No. 10 was at Christmas and would arrange for me to revisit with my mum, sister and friends just two months later. It, and the many trees that could light a whole neighbourhood within the house, were indeed twinkly and lovely but it was also *absolutely ridiculous* that I was in that house *again* for the *third* time in two months. In later years I would find myself there twice more, but I never met the cat. Who knew that a cancer diagnosis meant you essentially move into No. 10, though? Anyway. I'm jumping ahead.

The Pride of Britain Awards were televised the same week as our trip to No. 10 for the Breast Cancer Awareness Month reception. I was so nervous to watch the awards back, dreading what people might say and the wave of sympathy that might be about to drown me. I wanted people to see me as a woman on a mission, not the poor bald girl with cancer. I wanted people to see the energy I had garnered throughout those months, not the cancer victim. I guess it would have been handy if they'd known me before all this, but only I did, so really only I knew and saw what others never could. Whatever happened, we needed to ensure our website was up and running in time for the show. The awards became a sort of national launch of the charity – suddenly people would have heard of CoppaFeel! It was advertising we could never pay for and MAN, did we want to maximise this opportunity.

The show aired. We were in London. The next morning I remember walking down the street with my friends and family and I heard a woman shout, 'You're inspirational!' out of her car window. Usually you wouldn't bat an eyelid at people yelling or shouting something in a big city, but the day after being on TV I was unnervingly aware of my presence in the world (I didn't yet know if I liked that feeling or not). I stopped to look around at who she might be shouting at before realising she was looking at me. I was so embarrassed, yet I smiled, nodded and said thanks. What the hell was happening? Later that day, as I met a friend for lunch at Borough Market, someone stopped me to tell me they'd seen the show last night and wanted to wish me well.

The emails and messages of support on our Facebook group flooded in from all over the country, and some from even further afield. One chap from Verbier in France told me he was going to organise a fundraiser for Coppa-Feel!, and there was another message from an adventurer who had just rowed across the Indian Ocean and by chance had tuned in to the show last night and felt compelled to write. Others wanted to thank me for coming on stage without a wig. Not much thinking went into that decision – I just couldn't be arsed to wear it – but little did I know it would help a woman I'd never met feel confident to not wear hers around her children. There were some creepy admirers, *many* links to so-called 'wonder cancer cures', but on the whole a barrage of loveliness. It was exhausting. But I was buzzing. I wanted to bottle up that feeling I was experiencing; I wanted to hand it to everyone else with cancer, see if it might just make them feel better too. My hair sprouted twice as fast in those few exciting days, I'm sure of it.

*

When the Breast Cancer Awareness reception evening arrived, ten of my friends and I sauntered into the place like we were off to a mate's house for a knees-up. We'd all rushed there from various places and I remember Maren's boyfriend Graham having to get changed in a telephone box near Big Ben like Superman, as he'd only managed to get to London from Cornwall with seconds to spare. I did not want to be late – how would that look? I, of course, was most confident out of all of us, as I'd only been there two weeks earlier, the day after the awards ceremony. I was so brazen I almost high-fived Gordon Brown when I saw him again. I loved my new-found cockiness. Apart from my ten mates, a.k.a. 'campaign colleagues', I knew no one there, as we were the new breast-cancer-world kids on the block.

I convinced myself that I was important enough to speak to. Breast cancer charity CEOs, MPs, campaigning groups and patient advocates were hobnobbing and probably using this opportunity very wisely, making connections and handing out business cards. We, on the other hand, had nothing but our stickers in one hand and some posh vino in the other. Our mission was for everyone to leave that event with a hand sticker on their chest. We'd already seen how receptive young people at festivals and celebrities at big fancy awards nights had been to this stunt, so surely some MPs and important-looking folk would be just as keen? Whether they were or not, they had little choice. My cheeky – but might I also add polite – pals won them over and I truly believe brightened up what would have probably otherwise been a dry evening (no offence, guys). I got to meet the hairdresser Trevor Sorbie, who had been providing free wig hairstyling for cancer patients. I was introduced to Sarah Brown, wife to Gordon (and awesome woman in her own right); she was so friendly and kind and made me feel so comfortable.

I make out like this was all really normal and natural, but of course my palms and pits were sweaty. Hot flushes from the chemo were my pal by then and I'd developed a leaky left eye as a side effect too, so yeah, I probably didn't look all that calm and collected. But I never wanted to forget how this all felt: that I wasn't out of my depth, that we did belong there. Sarah Brown calmed me. Whether she meant it or not, she was keen to tell me that if there was anything we might need help with, I shouldn't hesitate to ask. I thought for a second and then remembered that we'd heard nothing from the Charity Commission about our application. We'd sent off the paperwork, expected to wait a while, but the silence made us worry whether we'd maybe been unsuccessful. I've no doubt she wasn't expecting me to take up her offer there and then or (possibly/hopefully) ever, but before I or she could prepare, out of my mouth came, 'Well, you could check up on whether we are getting charity status or not.' She paused. 'Absolutely, leave it with me.' Her assistant scribbled notes on a pad of paper. *Cool*, I thought.

From that day on I've always vowed to take people up on their offer of help, whether you think they mean it or not – you'll soon find out when their hand is outstretched or there's silence. We were the last bunch to leave the event, not before grabbing the opportunity for some cheeky shots of us pretending to be PM by the front door – oh and sticking a CoppaFeel! hand next to the figure 10. I mean, seize the day and every opportunity, right?

Again, as we made our way back to Maike's flat in South London (a place I had been staying at rather a lot that summer, what with hobnobbing in London all of a sudden), I couldn't help but wonder who this new Kris was. How had she got so confident? How was she now so resolutely sure of herself and her new mission? Did the wine help? Maybe. Did she just feel like she had nothing to lose? Probably. Did it all go to her head a bit? Definitely.

You know those times when you are so unsure of yourself you morph into something else. You are so plagued by fear of judgement that you hide behind yourself. That's how I felt for approximately 80 per cent of the time before I was diagnosed. There was this time in Beijing at a lunch meeting with some colleagues (one older, one younger, seemingly wiser) when I couldn't accept who I was or see how I was going to change it. When we weren't discussing all the weird things that were occurring in the city around the time of the Olympics (i.e. dogs larger than a certain size disappearing or the fact it was sunny, without fail, every weekend), conversations, as is normal, sometimes moved on to topics I knew nothing about. Such as philosophy. It's tricky when you hear the words 'favourite philosopher' and your only thought is the Natasha Bedingfield lyrics about Byron and Keats – and they're poets, not philosophers. I already felt quite inferior to my colleagues, but this gave me a whole new level of self-torment. I didn't know any of the names of the philosophers they were talking about or their theories – maybe I should have taken that sixth-form critical-thinking class I thought was such a 'doss' after all? I so badly wanted to have someone else's brain for just, like, an hour, so I could feel like I belonged. Instead of admitting I knew nothing (which would have been absolutely fine) I pretended the opposite and sat there nodding, agreeing to theories and views and opinions that were not my own. I mean, I didn't even have my own! I couldn't trust my own thoughts and so I stole others'.

This happened a lot. I would go home and cry because I felt useless and pointless. I felt I had *nothing* to offer anyone or anything, ever. It's dramatic, I know, and really the only reason this plays on my mind now, when maybe it should just be left in the 'you were young, it can be forgiven' archives, is because of the contrast in my attitude and confidence not that long after. The only difference was a life-threatening diagnosis; I hadn't suddenly become well read and well clever. I had just become comfortable in my own skin and brain. (And in fact, at that lunch meeting in the blistering heat that day in Beijing, I already had cancer – I just didn't know it.)

The morning after the reception at No. 10 I received a call. I didn't file to memory where exactly I was, who I was with, only what I was hearing.

'Hi, it's Fred from Downing Street.' That was definitely not his name. But it was undoubtedly a bloke.

'I've just looked into your application with the Charity Commission and they have reassured me that you will hear from them soon.' I surely remember those words well.

'Cool,' I think I said. 'Thank you,' I definitely said. Trying not to squeal or cry – or both.

Coming back down to earth after a whirlwind couple of weeks was hard. I'd been picked up by a tornado and plopped back out, back at Mum's, back to the reality of cancer. Something that helped quell my sudden drop in adrenaline was the addition of a new kitten that I named after a Japanese anime heroine, Princess Mononoke. Noke for short nowadays. I needed her playful distractions and silliness (but definitely didn't need her to scratch me, to bleed like crazy and panic that she'd given

me a horrible infection that might kill me. LOL, CATS!).
I also had a birthday party to plan just two months later,
Maren's and my twenty-fourth at the top of St Thomas's
Hospital funded by the amazing Willow Foundation
(those lovely folk who organise special days for people
with terminal illnesses), at which, naturally, I dressed as
Princess Mononoke.

People were really good to us. After my appearance on
the *Pride of Britain Awards* complete strangers would
share their own cancer stories with us, declare they were
going to take on a big challenge in aid of us, or even, like
one young girl called Fran, shave their head. There was,
and still is, a constant flow of love, admiration and
encouragement that became as vital to me as the air I
breathed. I needed the reassurance we were doing
something good, that all the hard work was worth it. I
would always be thinking that maybe someone,
somewhere, had found the courage to speak to their GP
because of us.

One-Tit Wonder

BLOG POST, SOMETIME 2009

It's hard to explain to all non-cancer folk, but this 'trip' I'm on gets kinda tedious every now and again. Imagine being on a train to an unknown destination and every time it approaches a new stop it slows down, and just when you think you could get out to admire the views, it speeds up again. You ask whether you can ever get off and all you get is blank looks. While I'm on this train to hell-knows-where, should I be checking out what snacks they sell in the food carriage, what cocktails the hot barman can whip up for me and whether someone wants to play a game of Shithead?

The time for my boob removal finally arrived. By that point a TV exec from the BBC had been in touch asking me to start documenting my life. She hadn't had any confirmation of a commission, but if that came we didn't want to miss the mastectomy featuring in it. Although, in the end, nothing came of it, calls like hers had begun to feel pretty normal. I'd done so many interviews that an email asking whether I'd consider filming my entire life and sharing it with the world didn't even faze me. A few nights before the operation, a friendly chap from the production team delivered a camera along with the book *The Power of Now* by Eckhart Tolle – odd (I had never met him before) but nice. We'd agreed Maren would film me meeting friends or looking vacantly into nothing, and we'd also been asked to do diary cams the night before the operation.

As I babbled away to the camera, I realised how I'd actually not had any time to really prepare. I mean, in physical time it had been eight months since my diagnosis, so you'd think I'd be more than ready. But I'd filled life with so much that I just never really gave it much thought. All I knew for sure is that I was glad to get rid of what felt like the source of the problem. I wanted to rid my body of the culprit. After months of radiotherapy and chemotherapy, I wanted that chapter to close. Sure, there were still many *many* chapters to come, but this one could be folded away. In fact, this is what I said the night before:

It's just dawned on me that I'm losing a part of me tomorrow. It's a part of me but it's not what defines me. It feels very strange, but this is all part of the process of fighting this beast and ridding [myself of] this bitch once and for all. I'm positive I'm making the right decision. I'm aware some doctors might think it's pointless having a mastectomy now when it's already spread, but I know I'm making the right decision, because I'm giving myself the best chance to beat this. *casually sips tea* All day people have been sending me messages wishing me luck, but I'm not sure this is a luck situation. I'd say I've been pretty bloody unlucky so far and it's not been on my side. So, I just want to get it over and done with now. It's time.

I would give both my breasts tomorrow if they knew for certain I was going to live for as long as possible, but who can know anything like that for certain anyway? Vanity shouldn't really come into play now. I've never felt very attached to my boobs, I've never really liked them, so why would I start liking them now that I'm losing one of them? This is probably (maybe?) going to be much easier than some of the treatments I've had to endure til now, and I'm going to be out of it for this one and on morphine for twelve hours as well, so that will be quite nice, and after that it will be about getting my arm moving again, I guess, from what I've understood.

I can do this. Someone I don't even know messaged me to say that I was 'infinitely more than a pair of breasts', so that's quite nice to know. It's reassuring to know that there's more to me than a pair of boobs. Apparently guys like bums anyway?

What can I say? I was profound. But seriously, did I need to be so strong? It's like I'd set the tone – upbeat and chirpy – for my way of dealing with cancer and I was *not* going to stray from it for *anything*. I don't recall being scared or fed up, but I can't say if that's because I buried that emotion so very deep that I have no memory of it now. Perhaps you can't feel what you can't allow? Either way, I know now it would have been just as OK to have howled my way through that video.

The morning we drove to the hospital I wasn't sure if I'd be returning home that day or not. It would all depend on how well the op went and how I felt coming round from the anaesthetic. Maren, Maike and Mum all accompanied me. I remember there being lots of waiting around, waiting for the surgeon to come and draw stuff on my boob with felt tip (ensuring they chop the right one off), waiting around for a nurse to come and take my vital stats, waiting around to finally get the call that it was time to go to theatre. I don't remember being scared then either. I don't remember feeling much, but I do remember that wearing the hospital gown made me feel like a patient for the very first time – my logic being that if I looked like a sick person, I would be a sick person.

Nine months before I might have worried a lot more, but the Kris I had morphed into knew it was going to be OK. To be honest, apart from dying during the operation, I wasn't sure what I should be worried about. In my head I already existed without two boobs, right from the day I was diagnosed on 19 Feb, when they had told me this would happen. Back then they expected it to take place within a week, but here I was, eight months down the road. It was more than time. 'Get this bloody thing off me,' I vaguely remember saying, before counting back from ten as the anaesthetic kicked in.

I was groggy when I came to. I felt hot, sore, like I'd been dragged along a road under a car, on my front, over barbed wire. I had, thankfully, been given my own room in the hospital to rest. I looked down at my chest and winced in pain. I couldn't make out if the boob was successfully gone, but I assumed, with all the bandages around me and the drainage tube hanging out of me (to collect excess fluid that can accumulate in the space where the tumour has been), that it probably was. The nurses reassured me that it had gone to plan. I was in and out of sleep, the morphine was doing its job, but my mouth was drier than the sun and I was desperate for water.

I don't remember how long it was until my family was allowed to see me, but eventually, coming back round from a nap, I saw Maren like an apparition. She was muttering something that included the numbers 1132366. It took me a little while to understand that she was telling me our charity registration number. She was telling me that we had, on that day, 28 October 2009, been granted charity status. That moment only really became significant on reflection. There I was, recovering from an operation that was ridding my body of cancer, albeit not *all* the cancer, but at least the OG bully, and at precisely the same time something was about to begin. I must have tried really hard to muster the energy to show my elation. I remember feeling it, but it was probably really subtle at the time. I probably fell back to sleep within seconds.

The test I needed to pass before I was allowed to go home was whether I could walk to the toilet. I was far too weak and failed. They decided I should stay a night, give me time to rest, be checked up on by some lovely nurses and watch telly in my own room. As I lay in that bed in the hospital, I realised it was the very first time I had been on my own since my diagnosis. There wasn't a day or a night that went past that I didn't have a friend or family member nearby, and now here I was, completely alone. *Being alone is really great sometimes*, I thought. I was wired. Excited about Maren's news. The street lights outside cast a light on the walls that I became transfixed by. Eventually I must have drifted off.

OK, that is a blatant lie. Truth is, before I managed to sleep I was texting a boy.

I wasn't really sure how and if I'd ever meet someone again after my diagnosis, and to be honest, it was far from my mind. Dating became one of many unthinkables. I was starting to have a relationship with the most important person of all, and that was me. We were communicating for the first time in my life and I didn't need anyone to intercept or fill a gap. I was learning my priorities and boundaries and what mattered. Until, of course, I met someone with a cute face who, ya know, smiled at me. Timings just haven't ever been my forte, but I'm pretty sure no one can really know when it's a good time to fall in love after a terminal cancer diagnosis or actually *ever*, for that matter. Cute-face boy was also affectionately known as Catface because it was a plain fact that he had very feline features.

They say you meet someone when you least expect it – I met Catface at the very first festival we took Coppa-Feel! to. I'd given him a cursory glance – I was still human, after all. There was this unexpected magnetism, an unsettling closeness that completely startled me. We met during the days when I finally realised my life was worth fighting for, and whatever air of vibrance and sexy virtuousness I was giving off very cleverly must have helped disguise the fact I was lacking hair on my bonce (not that that should matter, but *ya know*) and also the small, tiny, unsexy fact that I was very, very unwell. I must have been beaming with life enough to convince him I was on the market, not about to die, and still dateable. He was a friend of a friend who had been roped in to volunteer with us, so was already well aware of my story and predicament, saving me the spiel.

I contacted Catface under the pretext of asking his professional advice. At first our chats were centred around the charity and how he could help make our website better. It was all very businessy and in no way flirtatious – unless talking Pantone colours are a turn-on (although, come to think of it, to some graphic designers they probably are). Charity chats soon turned to more chatty chats, which eventually turned into dates and sleepovers. Cancer can throw your trust and respect in your body off-kilter. It's incredibly hard to start an intimate relationship with someone with that mentality alone, before you add on the emotional baggage from my previous relationship. But he made me feel safe and desirable, even if I didn't feel it. He was the last person to see me with two boobs, in fact, and not just see but remind me of the sensual delights of my breasts, something that is swiftly forgotten after you find out your boobs want to kill you. He became a pretty great distraction and a handy place to stay in London.

Once my mastectomy was healed enough, I was prepped for radiotherapy on my chest. Fifteen sessions over fifteen consecutive days were lined up to try and zap up any leftover cancer cells the chemo and surgery might have missed from the primary breast cancer site. They'd managed to get enough 'clearance' of the area to be pretty sure they'd got it all, but nothing is more definitive than blasting the lot. The monotony of those visits became pretty draining. We were edging ever closer to Christmas and with that came the incessant festive music blaring out of the radio that the nurses had tuned in to. 'All I Want for Christmas' took on a whole new meaning. Just a year before I had been prancing around my apartment in Beijing with Aya, singing along loudly – and, admittedly, wincing every two seconds from the pain in my back. I actually recall Aya laughing at me for my pained moves. How vastly different life had become. Back then fearing the worst; now experiencing the worst, but with far greater excitement for the present and possible future.

The sessions turned my skin a dappled texture and gave me a perma-tan that lasted for about, I think, five years. I applied Sudocrem before bed every night, and before I knew it, the squishy post-surgery foob (my fake boob) was upgraded to a prosthetic one and I adjusted to life with my Cyclops boob. I can tell you it wasn't that different from life before. It was winter, so perhaps the fact that I didn't have to hide my new uneven chest helped me come to terms with it all, or perhaps I really just wasn't that bothered.

There seems to be some kind of unspoken insistence that when you have a breast removed it needs to be immediately replaced. However, I couldn't help but think that would be for other peoples' benefit, not mine. I didn't want to put something in my bra to fake an even chest. It's like no one is supposed to know the trauma I've been through. Nope. I'm not buying in to that. Audre Lorde wrote it so perfectly when she said that 'silence and invisibility lead to powerlessness' and I think we all know by now how I feel about being powerless. So if I am going to use a prosthetic it would be only to pad out a dress or top better, it certainly would not be to make my personal tragedies more palatable or satisfy the male gaze. Nowhere did I see any kind of celebration of a body that only had one boob around the time of my first mastectomy. (Eleven years later, after my elective mastectomy – meaning I CHOSE to have my healthy right boob removed for symmetry – my nurse arrived at my bedside with a plump and soft fake boob to put in my top for my hospital departure. I swiftly reminded her that I had just undergone the operation to be without boobs ON PURPOSE. It must have really challenged her very in-built view of 'normal'.)

As soon as the wound allowed, I carried on with regular swimming sessions, coached by a physio to help me regain full movement in my left arm. Having my entire lymph nodes removed from my left side made the tendons eyewateringly tight and I was adamant I'd nip that in the bud. It gave me yet more to focus on, a mini goal, something I could control.

The final few days of that life-altering year were spent many miles from home. On 28 December Maren and I stepped on a plane to California. I was doing something that I hadn't dared to believe was possible up until that very moment. I was doing something that pre-cancer Kris recognised: heading off on a trip away, abroad, international, many many miles from hospital and home. Away from everything that had just happened, and the anticipation of what might still be ahead of me. We put it all aside for some dreamy days with Aya and her family in Berkeley, camping on the coast at Point Reyes over New Year. Bringing in 2010 with fresh sea air in our lungs, fresh thoughts in our heads, bidding farewell to the year that had shaped a very new Kris. It allowed for some much-needed introspection and reflection of the last ten months. It allowed Maren and I to gather ourselves and be so very grateful.

No holiday or trip away had ever been SO doused in meaning. All my most recent trips abroad had been escapes, me trying to run away from myself, my existence, in search of something I didn't even know or would recognise if I found it. When the trip was over and we were sitting in the departure lounge at San Francisco airport, I felt something I'd *never* felt before: joy to be returning to my life. There was so much to look forward to: so many exciting ideas and opportunities whirring in my head constantly, a boy who genuinely seemed enraptured to see me again, and most of all a life I was happy to return to. It confirmed for me that travel was only ever an excuse to get outside of myself. Travel may have earned me money but not happiness. I mean, there was no way I'd ever know that for sure, but it was a relief that I could put the 'What if I hadn't got cancer?' questions to bed. There were no what-ifs; I only had what was certain: TODAY.

The Glitter

I didn't know when I'd finally realise that what I was doing – what we were pouring our hearts and souls into – made sense, impacted anything or anyone, and had some *real* meaning, but I never lost sight of the fact that that moment would come. I didn't know in what form, whether it would be physical or not, and I in no way anticipated it to be an email that popped into my inbox one chilly morning in January 2010.

Subject: Thank you . . .

Hi Kris,

I wanted to pop you an email as a great big thank you for getting your message across!! I read your article in Good Housekeeping *. . . here is my story for you. x*

*

I'm twenty-six years old, and after having a feel of the boobies one day in October, I found something that was unusual. So, as a good girl, I popped off to the doctor's . . . similar experience to you the first few times I went: 'too young to really be a risk', 'wait until your next period', etc. . . . until I read your article and showed it to my boyfriend, who promptly marched me off to the doctor's in the blizzards we were having at the beginning of January, with your article in hand. I said to the lady doctor again that I needed her to do something and I feel like I am not being taken seriously, I gave them three appointments already to do the right thing and help investigate, until I gave them no choice.

So off to the hospital I went, feeling very proud of myself that I had enough in me to say no to the doctor and push to see a consultant. I had an ultrasound and they did a shockingly unexpected biopsy (ouch), so good news, it appeared to be fibroadenoma (breast mouse! – benign) but I was to wait a week and come back in for the results. So on Monday this week I drove to the doctor's with my boyfriend, not really thinking about anything apart from what time I'd get to work and what to have for lunch, but with the gross feeling that I was going through the same steps that some ladies go through and it's bad news for them. The consultant checked me again. 'Only a little one,' he said, then sat down and explained that although last week they suggested it was a fibroadenoma lump, it was in fact bad news and I have breast cancer . . . you know my reaction . . . I, me, twenty-six-year-old me has cancer . . . (ooo here come the tears). Although I did say I felt like Kylie Minogue . . . to lighten the mood in the room.

Reading your story and learning about CoppaFeel! before I received this news from the consultant has given me such amazing strength. I'm a strong, stubborn girl as it is, but I want to thank you soooo much for getting your message out there to girls that they need to take this seriously and CoppaFeel every now and again. if it wasn't for your article, I'm not sure I'd have gone back as soon as I did.

As you do, I have an amazing family, group of friends and the most perfect boyfriend a girl could ask for. But speaking to someone that knows the emotions I am dealing with at the moment is what will help more, I think.

So, tomorrow I am going to the Shelburne Hospital in High Wycombe for my lump to be removed, along with a couple of lymph nodes to check to see if it has spread. I am a little scared, *but have heard that the dye they will inject will make my wee blue for days, which in my humour I am finding hilarious (I'll feel like a lady Smurf!!).*

I can't thank you enough or think of a way to let you know how I appreciate what you have done and admire your strength. I am in awe. All I can think to do is to help you and your team, get involved in your activities and help you spread such a worthy and much-needed message to us girlies and their boobies!! My boyfriend is in training and will be finding a triathlon to complete and it will all be in the name of boobies and CoppaFeel!

My one concern at the moment is how my parents are handling the news: is there any advice you can give?!

Thank you, thank you, thank you!

I am scared, but as brave and strong as they come!!! Smile is back now; emotions are up and down at the moment.

I'm going to be in touch xxx

Jenny (boobie feeler!)

Whenever I'm asked about my proudest achievements, I will always talk, gleefully, about Jenny's email and how we went on to meet, how she went on to become one of our very treasured Boobette ambassadors and a friend, and how, ten years later, she went on to have two beautiful healthy babies. Jenny was the reason we didn't quit when it all felt so fucking hard in the early days. We didn't know how much we needed that email until it popped in my inbox. Jenny is the reason (among many more since) we still exist today and Jenny is the reason we can all know with complete certainty that there can be life way beyond cancer, and that we should all strive for that opportunity and hold on to that hope.

What we are, sadly, not saying is that this is always guaranteed, however. The sad truth is that some breast cancers, even when picked up at the earliest stage possible, do come back, and sometimes with a vengeance. There are no guarantees with anything in life and with a smart-ass like cancer in tow, you'll never know where you stand. That doesn't mean we live in fear, you hear me! We hold on to Jenny's story and all the other Jennys who've followed since.

Being Scared But Doing It Anyway

All the time I spent sharing my story with CRUK – from the TV ad to speaking at their big fancy events – resulted in me being offered a job. They were cooking up a huge breast cancer fundraiser and asked if I wanted to be part of the events team. Me, having a part-time job, in London, at the UK's biggest cancer charity. SURE. I guess my most recent activities and achievements worked just as well as a CV or polished LinkedIn profile, and so suddenly I found myself at a desk with a computer at their HQ in Lincoln's Inn Fields, Holborn. I had an ID card that got me in and out of the building. I had people to have lunch with, I had a diary to add meetings to, I had SO much to learn and absolutely no time for imposter syndrome.

While working on the event, I was getting an insight into the world of big charities, and they so kindly offered me all the know-how and time I could absorb in my post-chemo brain. I wanted to know everything, see everything, do everything. Obviously CoppaFeel! was way off the hundreds of staff they had and not quite at the millions of pounds raised per year, but every great organisation starts somewhere – the expert in anything was once a beginner, right? As I signed the employment contract I felt so proud that I was becoming someone who could be looked to for advice and ideas. Lingering in the back of my mind was a worry about how I'd split my time between CRUK and my own charity, but since CoppaFeel! wasn't able to pay me yet, I saw it as an amazing opportunity to work on becoming the best leader I could be for the charity, and at the same time start earning money again – the first time since the cash in hand I was getting teaching English in Beijing.

It was terrifying. I mean, almost everything about my life was new. But it wasn't life-threatening, and somehow cancer had made me brave enough to jump in the deep end, and so I told myself that unless the consequences might be death, I shouldn't let fear stand in my way. I was starting to see how cancer had forced me to recalibrate my relationship with change.

Taking this job forced Catface and me to turn the dial up on our relationship rather swiftly and all of a sudden I stayed at his house a lot. I'd wake early, walk from his flat in Clapham North to the Tube station, sit on the Northern line with everyone else who seemingly had some kind of purpose, start work at 9 a.m., finish at 5.30 p.m. and, try as I might, my heart just wasn't in it. I was learning loads and although fully committed to the task in hand, all I could think about was CoppaFeel! How could I do the work justice when I was only thinking about the future of my own charity? I couldn't help but think that any time not working on building CoppaFeel! was time wasted – and I was all too aware how precious a commodity like time for someone like me was. When the event I was working on was postponed, I saw it as an opportunity to part ways. I decided it was time to fully commit to CoppaFeel! Yes, that still meant being unpaid, and sure, I was as naive as ever, and I absolutely did cry like a baby when I told my line manager I was leaving, but my mind was made up.

Every idea for the charity was exciting; every possibility made something in my belly do a little backflip. You know when you can't sleep because an idea is keeping you wired and awake and there's no point in trying to sleep until you've at least fleshed it out on paper or on email or the notes app on your phone? This feeling would be what I would come to depend on time and time again; something that kept me fuelled and driven; a feeling I wished we could bottle up and share with other cancer patients; a sort of drug I had started to believe may just keep me alive. Of course, at times it was overwhelming and stressful too. I was impatient and basically wanted everything to happen overnight. I think the fact the charity had sprung from nothing in under a year only fed my need to continue on that same trajectory and ride that momentum.

I took on every opportunity that came my way. We'd organised our second CoppaFeel! half-marathon event at the Bath Half, I was signed up to do Race for Life and Walk the Walk, and we'd organised a bike ride in Cornwall with Olympic athlete Denise Lewis, all while not living in London, living out of a suitcase (Catface wasn't so keen on me taking up precious cupboard space) and keeping up with treatment back in Northampton. At a Mulberry sample sale in aid of CoppaFeel! one very hot and sunny day in Central London, I broke down. It had all got too much. Our organisation lacked the foundations it needed to sustain my energy and ensure I didn't burn out. We needed an office. We needed a team. And I needed a nap. But first I had a music festival to pull off.

In a dark, dingy, sticky-floored pub nestled on the Gray's Inn Road, hopping distance from King's Cross station, our very first Festifeel was birthed. With the help of our Australian friend Sarah (who Maren and I had met packing apples in Melbourne) and her boyfriend Liam, we put together a line-up of music, from acoustic bands to DJs, to fundraise and celebrate the start of another full summer of touring festivals. We'd started the charity in a field, surrounded by music, accompanied by the beat of a drum, and so it became part of our DNA. You wouldn't recognise most of the names on the line-up, but that didn't matter – we had created our very own event that people (OK, mostly friends) came to. Jenny and her boyfriend Gareth came; Simon, the chap who watched me on the telly and organised an event raising over £4,000 in Verbier, even MC'd.

Looking around, I saw the faces of the people who had believed in us or had in some way been affected by us, by my story. A story that on the surface was a pretty tragic one but had now spawned *this*. And although I recognised most of the faces in there now, I knew there'd be a time when I'd look around Festifeel and not know anyone. That I would have to guess their story instead of knowing it verbatim. That's when I'd feel really accomplished, I thought. That's when I'd know I was doing enough, that the charity had a future without me, that I could take one step away and observe rather than constantly *do*. I clung onto these future visions as we danced the night away to our headliner – someone you probably have heard of – Newton Faulkner, who I had met at one of the many CRUK events I gave a speech at. (What can I say? I'd got good at asking for help.)

Shortly after the success of Festifeel, I was beginning to realise that Catface had become more of a full-time designer for CoppaFeel! and less of my boyfriend. I was staying at his house more out of convenience than anything – and FYI, convenient is something a relationship should never be. This ultimately broke our communication and destroyed all the joy of those early days of silliness, of naughtiness, of discovering each other, of being in love. He eventually called time on our relationship on the basis of not really knowing what he wanted from 'us'. I was, once again, heartbroken, but could, unlike my previous relationship downfalls, see sense in it all – after I did a lot of ugly crying, of course.

I had also, unlike previous break-ups, a lot of things to distract me. I jumped straight into a writing job, telling the tales of my cancer life in a monthly column for my local paper – the *Northampton Chronicle & Echo* (and later for the *Mirror* before graduating to the *Sun*). By this point I was also being mentored by a hero of a woman called Kate Lee. She was the CEO of a hospice in Warwickshire and knew just about everything I could ever wish to know about leading an organisation, while also being a fun human and somehow seeming like she had her shit together. She became, and still is, my ultimate life, charity and CEO guru – at the time of writing she leads the Alzheimer's Society.

Kate spent many hours sitting with me, Maren and Jamie formulating a strategy. That was a word that was so new to me; I'd never so much as strategised the day ahead, let alone thought of the charity's life in any kind of sensible yearly plan. It was mind-boggling yet so reassuring. She made us imagine where we'd be, both with the charity and personally, in one year, three years, five years and even ten. She asked us how we'd sharpen the saw – in other words, how we'd ensure we'd always remember to have fun, which in turn would sustain and strengthen the resilience we would need when times got tough – oh, they would get tough – and make opportunities to simply breathe, take stock and celebrate even small wins.

Exit strategies were never danced around, and although mine wasn't so much retiring and more like dying, we decided we'd rename it 'When Kris goes to the Maldives'. We future-proofed the charity by future-proofing me. Kate helped us shape a robust charity and over the years came to my aid many times when I just didn't feel like I fitted into the boots of a charity CEO, always successfully calming and encouraging me. Literally anything was possible after a chat with Kate.

We led another jam-packed summer of festivals, this time with all the learnings from our first year, a few more paintbrushes, a better gazebo and some space hoppers (which once got stolen – we didn't notice until we saw them being catapulted onto the main stage at Beach Break Live). By the end of the summer I was happier, more settled again and somehow, realising that we did really really like each other and could definitely make it work, I got back together with Catface. You know how it is. OK, maybe you don't, but suffice to say being with him felt good again.

'I've decided I want to move to London,' I sheepishly announced to Mum one day. I had been dreading telling her, as I was worried about how she'd react. She'd become my carer for a year, seeing me through five months of gruelling chemotherapy, watching me recover from a mastectomy, start hormone drugs and get excited about CoppaFeel! She'd excelled and thrived in Mum mode. I'd absorbed her need to be needed when I was a kid. Then, when I was a teenager, unless she was driving us to friends' houses or picking us up from parties, she was 'superfluous to our needs'. This line landed sharply the first time, but once you hear it over and over again it kinda loses its impact. Maren and I thought we were doing what every young person does – becoming independent – but this didn't always suit Mum, and at times it made me want to rebel all the more.

Mum never met anyone else to spend the rest of her life with after Dad. She'd frown when we said we were heading out with our boyfriends or friends. I was aware of the void we created whenever we weren't around. So imagine having a sick daughter with cancer who has needed you more than ever for twelve months telling you she's moving out. She, like me, had probably never expected this day to arrive.

By this point I was already spending so much time in London, sleeping on friends' sofas, that it really just made sense. My friend Faye was moving to London and starting her job at John Lewis HQ at the same time, and since there was no way I could afford to live on my own in London, and not wanting to rush our relationship and move in with Catface, sharing with Faye was a perfect solution. I found a flat online, and although it was way more than either of us could afford, I was adamant that living somewhere that didn't smell of mouldy residue or was the size of a matchbox was paramount. Obviously the fact it was on Copperfield Street played absolutely no role whatsoever! I used some of the Disability Living Allowance I received for having terminal cancer (finally granted to me after my GP signed a 'special rules' form on which she had to say that I'd likely be dead in six months. That was a nice chat) along with inheritance.

Five hundred and seventy days after hearing, 'You have incurable cancer,' I was spending my first night in an apartment with a tenancy agreement with my name and six months' rent on it. I was allowing myself to believe in a future that stretched beyond my usual limit of, say, one week. Planning far ahead never came naturally to me, even before a terminal diagnosis – a fact that very likely helped with the roadblocks cancer put in my way – but now I was placing some tentative faith in the future.

As I lay in my bed, surrounded by a select few belongings from home, I settled into the idea that life was panning out OK. I mean, I had already made it this far: I'd established a charity that was garnering more and more attention each day, my cancer was under control with the help of Tamoxifen and a bone-strengthening monthly infusion called Zometa, and I now lived in an apartment in Mile End with a balcony overlooking a river lock (and a park you wouldn't want to walk through at night, but let's stick with the positives) with my oldest school friend. I'd still have to pop back to Northampton General Hospital for the infusions, but that was the compromise of trying to get on with life *and* actively working on staying alive. I'd either head home the evening before the appointment so I could spend some time with Mum or try and wedge my infusions into a one-day round trip if I had 'too much on'. It's amazing how flexible and doable anything can be when your life depends on it.

A lot of CoppaFeel!'s noteworthy moments tend to stem from one event. The nucleus, the catalyst that led to more good stuff: the Pride of Britain Awards. We have my (still unworthy but OK, OK, I will accept it) win to thank for so many things: one was us landing desk space in a red-brick building, smack bang in the middle of Clerkenwell, with its many fancy coffee shops and mini Waitrose. A chap I'd been introduced to, and fellow winner, named Phil Packer, was true to his word when he said, 'Let me know if I can ever help with anything. Let's stay in touch.' I stayed in touch. And I asked for help. 'Don't suppose you know anyone with a spare desk somewhere in London that wouldn't mind us setting up a little CoppaFeel! Boob Hive as we work on world domination, etc.?'

It was a long shot. Office space in London usually has a massive price tag and at this point no number of cake sales or raffles would cover the cost of a Central-London HQ. 'Actually, yes, I have an idea,' came his reply. I've always known the notion that if you want something, work hard and you shall receive. It's a nice idea, but it's ultimately bullshit. So much also depends on random circumstances.

He'd been working with an architects' practice called BDP, which was offering pro bono help with a purpose-built centre for residential trips for kids who needed help. I mean, he did win a Pride of Britain award for a reason. He kindly introduced me to the top dude, the dude with the power to say yes, the CEO, Peter Drummond. Before we knew it, Maren (who by this point had given up her garden-design career to work full time, unpaid, on Coppa-Feel!, still living in Cornwall but spending a vast amount of time with me in London) and I were tapping away on laptops at desks surrounded by busy working people, sipping our coffees – something I just decided I liked one day – and eating the subsidised food from the canteen served up by the happiest of guys called Robert. When you're a charity or, in fact, any start-up, and at the very foothills of it all, you are grateful for just about any leg-up. Not only did we get free desk space and access to meeting rooms (for an initial month that turned into three years) but also free postage and free printing. At times I looked around the open-plan office, imagining everyone there was working for CoppaFeel!, not designing outside play areas or fancy housing developments. I could picture what a busy office full of boob chat could look like and it didn't seem impossible. Although I didn't really believe that it took hundreds of people working across four floors of a huge building in Central London to get shit done – we'd already debunked that myth – it was becoming obvious that to build on all the successes and say yes to opportunities, we needed to invest in more man (or girl) power.

We'd made big plans for our first official Breast Cancer Awareness Month as a charity. We were still the new kids on the block and we needed to make a noise. We wanted to invest in our very first bit of media-campaign work and so, with the help of a pro bono ad agency named Archibald Ingall Stretton – our link being Steve Stretton, who promised to make a substantial donation to Coppa-Feel! if he got a mention in this book – we developed Boob Hijack. The idea: to hijack anything that looked like boobs with a sticker.

Back at that initial meeting about CoppaFeel! at Mum's we'd talked about speaking to students and setting up some kind of brand ambassador scheme. It made sense to target a group of people who were among peers who all needed to hear our message. Of course we wanted to speak to everyone (my mind was always 5 million steps ahead), including those who also didn't go to uni (after all, I hadn't!). But, one . . . step . . . at . . . a . . . time. We'd train them up about breast health – all the stuff we'd learned over the past year – set them some tasks that involved awareness as well as fundraising, and then let them get on with it. We'd let them show off their own creativity and a sense of autonomy, as ultimately they knew their student body and their campus culture better than us.

We employed the help of a student marketing company, which would recruit our student ambassadors. Signing our very first *paid for* contract with a supplier was momentous. All the fundraising efforts by countless wonderful humans (including our mega-old next-door neighbour David, who handed me our very first cheque for £100) for over a year had led to this day. Obviously we were investing in something we didn't know would work. The instincts we'd trusted, which had paid off thus far, were reassuring, but this was still scary. The company found and recruited fifteen amazingly enthusiastic students – some of whom we are still friends with today – and ultimately shaped the way we speak to young people. I felt like a mama duck proudly watching her ducklings head off on the big lake of life without her. I loved knowing that we were giving people the opportunity to do something potentially life-saving. The pressure and power no longer just lay with us. It wasn't just students who spread the word round their campuses – we asked the nation to join in too. I ended up hijacking Lorraine Kelly's boobs live on TV and projecting a huge image on to the *Angel of the North*. We marched around London chanting about boobs, asking people to check theirs. Madness.

Then came another pant-shitting-scary decision: we were going to take the plunge and employ someone. The power of TV brought a Kiwi named Dom into our lives. Having witnessed her sister go through cancer and leading a very successful 'don't drink and drive' campaign for young people in New Zealand, she had all the right credentials we needed. It was a big ask, on her part, to work alongside Maren and me (*twins*), being the first outsider and the first to be paid. Dom had to be capable of everything from strategic decisions to boring postal jobs and petty cash. And I was new to management. I've no doubt that even now the staff at CoppaFeel! would use very glowing words to describe my assiduous attention to detail, my commitment to authenticity and all the other terms we have that mean 'control freak'.

At twenty-four, I was the boss. I never thought of myself as a leader because I didn't like the picture it painted in my head, and probably yours too. I knew I held influence and I knew my passion could rub off on people and ignite the same level of energy, so I tried to harness all that without making myself seem too 'big'. I had all the credentials I needed but wore them lightly – at least, that was the plan. I could see myself as a visionary, which might sound grandiose, but I had big ideas, and could see a world in which people didn't die of breast cancer because their cancer was found late. I also wanted to be liked, but I didn't really know then that liking someone and working well with them aren't necessarily the same thing, and if you want to make things happen the latter is actually way more important. I was still in the early days of working out who I was becoming and how this new-found role fitted me.

I was also forced to question how much of the Cancer Kris I should let spill over into being a boss. Although the charity had started with my story, I had every intention of keeping work and cancer separate to try and maintain whatever authority I had garnered, and to seem, at least to some degree, professional. I would soon discover that although this was a nice idea, it could never work in reality – cancer was the real boss, not me; cancer made the schedule, however much I fought it.

He-Man

We were now a thriving charity with three official full-time staff – me, Maren and Dom – and it was a fairly ordinary day at Boob HQ. Maren was in London, which meant we were probably cramming in seeing anyone and everyone to make the most of her time in the Big Smoke. During a weekly meeting with our volunteer fundraising manager, Beth, I felt my back twinge out of place. As I had tied my shoelaces earlier that morning something hadn't felt quite right in my lower spine, but like any other pain, I was able to shrug it off.

I had come to recognise that if I were to freak out about any ache or pain in my body, I'd never get anything done. I would assess the situation with: can I walk and can I sit at a desk and do work? (The only real cause for alarm was if I had no appetite. Much like when a cat doesn't eat, it means it's preparing to die, I always fear(ed) the same for me.) If I could answer yes to those questions I wouldn't bother my mind too much with what-ifs. But this pain graduated from a 'what if' to a 'definitely something not right' very swiftly in the dining hall that busy lunchtime. I yelped and alerted Maren and Beth to my new lack of ability to move. This pain felt like nothing I'd ever experienced. It was very different from any pain from the lower spine tumours just before I was diagnosed, which were subsequently zapped with radiotherapy. I lurched forward in agony. This was awkward. This was terrifying. This was embarrassing.

Maren and Beth thought it was probably best to call an ambulance but decided to wait until the lunchtime rush had calmed so as not to cause a massive scene. Whatever was happening with my skeletal system, I was more than happy to avoid the drama and worried faces. Two paramedics and a special chair contraption eventually appeared at my side. Given my current cancer status, they were in no way up for testing my movement for fear of making it worse. I needed pain drugs, pronto.

After an uncomfortable manoeuvre into the ambulance, I was swiftly hooked up to laughing gas and whatever else they were able to give me to numb the pain. I instantly felt better and suddenly quite chatty. I proceeded to tell the lovely paramedic lady (who would, GET THIS, after my little trip in her ambulance run a half-marathon for CoppaFeel!) my whole life's history when all she'd probably asked me for was my date of birth. I glanced over at Maren for reassurance but I got none. This was the first time in over two years that I had seen her strength falter. Her face said that losing me was not an option. But dying wasn't an immediate threat – it never really is with cancer – it's more that you go through stages of awareness of death, from mild to acute; 'it's OK' to 'shit's got real'. I gestured for her to take a drag of the gas and air too. I was reminded of our respective roles in this situation: she the powerless spectator, me the one who had to be prodded and poked.

The ambulance drew up at Barts Hospital and I went through all the usual A&E admission hubbub before finding myself in my own private room on a ward. No one was really sure what was happening and why. One thing we did consider is that I was still recovering from a vertebroplasty – a procedure where four pins were drilled into my spine to inject cement to stabilise and strengthen the vertebrae that were crumbling after being zapped so aggressively with radiotherapy two years earlier. Yup, it's as horrific and brutal as it sounds.

It had taken some time, after my oncologist requested this treatment, for the referral from Leicester Hospital to come through, but eventually I had been given an appointment with Dr Cement, a consultant musculoskeletal radiologist, who would be carrying out the torture. So, one hot and sweaty summer day Mum picked me up from the train station and took me to my appointment, thinking I would simply be talked through the operation, which I had already done potentially too much Google and YouTube-video research on, surprised I was OK for it to still go ahead.

I was taken into a room with Dr Cement, accompanied by the usual entourage of nurses, who brought in a chair for Mum to sit on (I hope my obsession with consultation seating arrangements hasn't gone unnoticed, guys). He began as specialists usually do, by looking at my referral letter from my oncologist, alongside my most recent scan images.

'I've looked at these images and can see you need some help stabilising those vertebrae that were treated with radiotherapy, but from what I can make out, I am not sure whether you actually had cancer in your lower spine in the first place.'

What?

OK. You might need to hold my wine for a second as I take you through this.

What he thought he saw on all the pictures that had been taken of my lower spine (L3–L5, to be precise) between February 2009 and now were not cancer cells but something called a haemangioma. At first my brain conjured an image of actual He-Man before quickly moving on to the fact that this man was telling me I might not even have advanced, stage 4, secondary breast cancer. On the basis of looking at a scan. With his eyeballs.

He went on to explain that a haemangioma was a sort of blood clot, a collection of blood cells all clustered together, like penguins when they huddle together for warmth in a snowstorm (that was not his explanation – it's mine). That what he saw on the scan might not be cancer, but blood. He couldn't be sure, of course – I mean, why be sure about these sort of things before letting them leak from your brain to your mouth, and then fly to my ears and swiftly on to my brain, which was at this point close to combustion – but he was keen to conduct a biopsy of the maybe-not-cancer while he was carrying out the cement work.

Afterwards Mum and I sat in her car in silence before I probably uttered 'what the fuck'. What the fuck. And one more time for good measure: what the fucking fuck. The thing is, he didn't need to plant this seed in my head at all. He could have simply explained that he was doing a biopsy – it's actually quite useful to have a sample of your cancer so you can check its latest hormone status or other clever, useful things that determine future treatment options – and waited until he knew more. I would just have nodded and agreed and been none the wiser. He didn't have to let me question what the hell my last two years had been all about. He didn't have to leave me feeling a bit sick and a bit faint on the train-station platform where Mum left me after the appointment as I made my way back home to London. He didn't have to put wild thoughts in my head that went a bit like this:

Kris, imagine if you don't actually have metastatic cancer. How do you explain that to the world? Will people think I'm a massive fraud? Will I be vilified like those people you hear about in the Daily Mail *who fake having cancer so they get loads of money donated for treatment and then fuck off to the Bahamas? Except I'm not in the Bahamas. I'm in fucking Leicester.*

I had just adjusted to this life; I had come to terms with the whole limited-life thing. This threatened my new identity. I didn't want anyone to take that away from me.

OK. Stop. WHAT ARE YOU SAYING?

This is the best possible news ever. Why aren't you doing cartwheels?

Man, I can't handle change. Wait. Hold on. I have had back pain since I was a kid. I saw an osteopath when I was twelve, who told me I'd have issues with my back when I'm older. My friend, who'd known me for six years, always told me my back is 'fucked'. I put my back out when I vommed in Beijing, so maybe that's when the fracture happened and this He-Man could have been the catalyst all along. It's plausible. Especially since they never did a biopsy when I was first diagnosed two and a half years ago; they only assumed the mass was malignant.

OK. I was starting to like this guy's thinking. Maybe he's inadvertently giving me the 'Get out of jail free and run away as fast as you bloody can' card. Maybe, just maybe, I no longer have cancer and I don't actually belong in the Stage 4 Club.

HOLY SHIT.

Being in my head was exhausting: I was imagining every scenario. I had to try so hard to think about anything *but* what he'd just said because until I got the results nothing had really changed. Except in my head everything had. It was cruel and unnecessary and, crucially, *really* inconvenient. We were about to get ready for our biggest Breast Cancer Awareness Month yet and the last thing I needed was *this*. (Yeah, OK, I know what you're thinking.)

Except that now, one month later, I found myself in Barts Hospital with a kind doctor's finger up my bum to rule out spinal compression. I've had my fair share of awkward, but this trumped (wrong choice of word?) it all. As I lay there, trying to calm my breathing and think of nice things, I can confirm that nothing, absolutely *nothing* can take your mind off the fact a complete stranger has inserted a digit into your arsehole. Guys, you might think that in the great scheme of things, what with everything else I'd had to endure up until then, that this would be something I'd handle OK. Nuh uh. I decided it was never OK for a finger to be inside my bum. The upshot was that I could tense my anus well enough to confirm my spine was still in working order. But I needed an MRI scan and X-ray to be sure.

Some time passed before I got taken for either scan. I was checking emails and fretting about work to pass all the minutes and hours in between. I hated whenever cancer interfered with anything to do with CoppaFeel!. As hard as I tried to never allow it to wriggle its way into my life as a charity boss, sometimes I'd have to admit defeat. Until they were sure my spine was OK, I wasn't going anywhere.

Sure enough, once the MRI and X-ray report was in, the doctors were happy for me to be discharged. The mild steroids and painkillers they pumped me with allowed me to move again and very slowly walk out of the hospital. They hadn't established why exactly I was in so much pain; they only ruled out any potential serious injury. The more day-to-day cancer stuff they handed back over to my medical team in Northampton.

Once my oncologist was up to speed with my latest adventures, he called me. He now had the results from the biopsy taken during the vertebroplasty and the full report of yet another scan. He hit me with a triple whammy of news: the mother of all cancer updates. Not only was Dr Cement, you guessed it, wrong, but the most recent scan from Barts Hospital showed I now had new cancer in my pelvis, my hips and also my liver.

'I'm so sorry,' he said. He was sorry too that I had been taken down a fantasy garden path of thinking I might not have metastatic cancer. He was bewildered by Dr Cement's unnecessary and now horrendously wrong assumption.

The news could not have been worse and yet suddenly the train I had been on for two years was back on its tracks. I'd worked so hard to suss this new life out and, aside from the fact I now had extra cancer to deal with and that my current cancer treatment was not sufficient any more, I felt safer simply knowing the full picture again. It seems that's all I ever really want and need: full transparency, no bullshittery, and zero hesitancy. And any action-hero man who could be my lost third twin probably shouldn't be dicking around in my body anyway.

Later that day I saw my oncologist face to face. He was visibly disappointed that I had been through such emotional fuckuppery but was keen to tell me a plan of action. He also asked if I wanted to see the scan that showed my liver tumour. I shrugged and grunted. I didn't really know what to expect to see. I guess maybe something pretty monstrous, eating its way through one of my terribly important organs, having a feast, looking a bit angry, perhaps with horns? But nope. I had to squint and adjust my eyes to see what he was trying to show me: a patch of slightly darker grey on an already quite grey blob that was my liver. This tiny little innocuous patch. Cancer was still such a mystery to me. The way it finds fuel to grow, the way it can evade some of the most toxic drugs in the world, I couldn't help but respect it in some strange way. Contrary to how I would perhaps speak about it back then, I don't hate it. It's housed in my body, it's part of me; hating it would mean hating myself – something I vowed I'd stop doing after breaking up with Dan. To get through this my body would need all the love and respect it could get. My oncologist reminded me how ginormous my liver was, that there was still way more of the healthy section in comparison and that this little slice of doom wasn't going to be affecting my liver function, at least not yet. I was OK. I had heaps to think about in terms of treatment options but I was OK.

Something was telling me that my time at Northampton Hospital was up. At an event I'd recently attended with one of (a.k.a. our only) major donors (a.k.a. rich person/ legend who very generously and unceremoniously donates big dollar to worthy causes), I recalled being introduced to a top oncologist – I mean, isn't it funny when that happens? How potentially heroic people are just plopped into your life like that and then, ya know, happen to become the people that help you stay alive? Wild, isn't it?

I rifled through my wallet and fingered my way through all the business cards I'd been collecting. My business cards were my life. Every single one of them had the potential to propel CoppaFeel! a few steps forward. I cherished everyone I was meeting and anyone who pressed a card into my hand. I found the card for Dr

Hope (as a friend called him) and sent an email. I got a response almost immediately, saying to make an appointment with his secretary and come see him ASAP. I was not expecting such a swift reply, but within twenty-four hours I was sitting in his office on Harley Street, going through the options my current oncologist was offering.

Yes, they'd been great at providing me with 'gold standard' care in Northampton General Hospital, but I needed more than that now. Plus, Dr Hope was offering to treat me through his NHS clinic at Charing Cross Hospital in London, which meant I could stop my arduous trips back and forth to Northampton. Best of all, he wasn't keen to get too aggressive with treatment just yet. I can't tell you the feeling of relief when he said that while the cancer had outsmarted my current treatment, nothing suggested it was running away from us yet. We opted for a combination of letrozole, Zoladex and Faslodex – the triple endocrine (hormone) therapy combination he favoured. Although really bloody painful to administer, I would take the Zoladex (a ridiculously large needle inserted into belly blub) and Faslodex injections (inserted into your love handles) and swallow the letrozole pills over chemotherapy IV any day. I also went on to have radiotherapy on those not-at-all-He-Man-like cancerous tumours residing on my spine.

Epic-Genetics

In recent years we have tried to discover why I got cancer and Maren didn't. We are identical, monozygotic beings (we came from the same fertilised egg, which split very early in the pregnancy), sharing the same genes and DNA. Our pals at the Twin Research Centre in London, specialists in a clever thing called 'epigenetics', have helped us understand this a little more. What was it about my cells that made them decide to go off-piste, and what is it about Maren's that makes them not? I was tested for the breast cancer gene mutations they currently know about not long after my diagnosis. A positive result for the commonly known BRCA mutations would mean Maren's chances of getting breast cancer were over 80 per cent. The fact that Maren might be predisposed to cancer too was very much an afterthought for her (have I told you how great and selfless she is?). The test came back negative, Mar got to keep her boobs and for now receives annual MRI scans to ensure that any abnormalities are picked up at the earliest point possible.

Epigenetics refers to external modifications to our DNA that turn genes 'on' or 'off'. At some point in my life, my environment, stress levels, diet or other lifestyle factors could have changed how my cells read some genes. The father of twin research and epigenetics at King's College, Professor Tim Spector, is fascinated not by the similarities in twins, but by the differences. He once quizzed me on our childhood for one of his (many) books: when my periods started, how I coped with our parents' divorce, what my diet was like. The only thing we could pinpoint was how differently Maren and I reacted to life and change as kids. The way I handled emotions and stress growing up was different from Mar. I stewed long and hard over Mum's happiness, over friendships, over schoolwork, over being a good girl, never wanting to disappoint. Maren, on the other hand, seemed to take things much more in her stride. I internalised it all. Something was different about the way we responded to stress. I know for a fact Maren noticed the same things I did but a traumatic event is only traumatic if it's experienced as such.

Doctor, author and legend Gabor Maté explains the connection between emotion and illness better than I ever could in his book *When the Body Says No*:

Stress is a complicated cascade of physical and biochemical responses to powerful emotional stimuli. Physiologically, emotions are themselves electrical, chemical and hormonal discharges of the human nervous system. Emotions influence – and are influenced by – the functioning of our major organs, the integrity of our immune defences and the workings of the many circulating biological substances that help govern the body's physical states. When emotions are repressed, this inhibition disarms the body's defences against illness. Repression – dissociating emotions from awareness and relegating them to the unconscious realm – disorganises and confuses our psychological defences so that in some people these defences go awry, becoming the destroyers of health rather than its protectors.

Our brains are so powerful! OK so for example, imagine Haribo Tangfastics (if you don't know what they are, then imagine a sour lemon) – now notice what your mouth has done. It's produced saliva, hasn't it? And that's all because you *imagined* something sour in your mouth. Similarly, if you were confronted with something horrific right now, maybe a child screaming in fear, you would notice that your heart rate rises, but then there would also be stuff you wouldn't notice, such as your digestion stopping, your hormone balance shifting – it's the physiological changes that we can't see that might be having the deepest long-term impact that can lead to cancer or other illnesses.

The relationship between breast cancer and stress has been researched a lot. A few studies of women with breast cancer* have shown a significantly high rate of disease among those who experienced traumatic life events and losses within several years before their diagnosis. Need I remind you of my toxic relationship? Gabor Maté also once wrote: 'When we have been prevented from learning to say No, our bodies may end up saying it for us.'

I can't say for sure that it's my childhood inner turmoil or the self-loathing caused by my relationship with Dan that caused havoc in my body (cancer is, after all, a multi-factorial disease and stress is just one contributing factor), and I would happily argue that it's those early childhood and teenage stressors that helped build the resilience I have to cope with cancer, but it makes me realise that cancer is not necessarily as random as we think. In the early days of my diagnosis I would hastily say that I was simply 'unlucky', but reading many books on the mind–body connection and lots of thinking (by me and way more clever people) has made me re-examine that.

---

* 'Psychological stress and breast cancer incidence', Valentina-Fineta Chirac, Baban, Adriana and Dumitrascu, *CLUJUL Medical*, 15 Jan 2018, https://www.ncbi.nlm.nih.gov/pmc/articles/PMC5808262

Knowing that doesn't necessarily change much for me now – other than contributing to my exploration as to how I, from here on out, deal with emotion and stress – but it's become a fascination and a journey of self-discovery for me to know what I may still have buried deep inside, and a lifelong commitment to let that shit go.

At the risk of sounding like a Gabor Maté fangirl (I am one) I wanted to add something he noted too. He is keen to point out that thinking about how our emotional responses are connected to our health issues is not about blame. It is not about saying, 'You didn't deal with your stress properly, so that's why you got x disease.' And this is absolutely not about pointing a finger at how I was parented, or my relationships (although, remember Dan wanted to own my cancer? I'm letting him, now. I'm good like that). 'Rather, it is about being honest with yourself from a lens of compassionate curiosity. It's about understanding that our physical health is intimately influenced by the level of health or stress within our psychological and social domains.'* Compassionate curiosity is my new favourite thing.

My hope is still that Maren and I can be of use to science, so we can understand why some people get cancer and others don't. But if we never find out why I have it, it won't matter. For me it's not so much about the

---

*   Gabor Maté

why – more about how I will deal with it, and with Mar with me I know I can. When the going gets tough, she puts the kettle on. When she lacks the words, she will instead find the necessary action. One time when I couldn't be consoled after bad scans, she flew our friend Georgette over from Sweden to cheer me up. If Georgette can't cheer me up, no one can. Mar isn't the sympathetic carer type; she's the one who will keep me grounded and will rarely even acknowledge I have cancer. She won't let me use cancer to my advantage unless it benefits her too – Blue Badge parking being a prime example. And this is exactly how I needed her, and still need her, to handle this. She says she takes her cues from me, so when I am positive, she is, and when I am sad she will likely be too.

Since my diagnosis our bond has grown stronger and it's no longer possible for me to fake anything around her. There was a time when I kept everything to myself for my own protection and to conceal a crippling sense of shame. I can't do that any more. I can't lie and say I'm fine when I'm in agony; I can't fake energy; I can't hide fear: she simply knows. She is my lie detector. Which is both useful, because she can help me without bringing it to anyone else's attention, and annoying because, well, it just is.

Life on Film

The sun had already made the inside of the van feel like an oven. I checked the time on my phone and it was still morning – how much hotter could today get? I yielded to the heat and lay on the squishy sofa after folding away the bed, listening to the distant galahs and not-so-distant crickets. We'd just finished breakfast outside and while everyone else was doing I'm not sure what, I grabbed the opportunity to finish Katie Piper's book *Beautiful*. I had heard of her story on the news or through social media, but in her own words her life became a wonder to me. I wasn't so into fiction – anything that didn't actually happen for real made it hard for me to connect with the words – but it was enthralling to read about other people's lives and how they traversed whatever turd that may have landed on theirs.

It was New Year's Day 2012 and I was feeling surprisingly fresh. We hadn't had too much to drink, or stayed up too late, even though I'd imagined/hoped for a romantic night gazing up at the stars with Catface. Alas, that didn't happen. At this point the cracks in our relationship were reappearing. But more on that later. Maren, Graham, Catface and I were parked up on a campsite walking distance from the beach, somewhere on the south-east coast of Australia. Our friends Sarah and Liam had just got married and so we used the wedding invite as an opportunity for a holiday too.

A nagging thought wouldn't leave me. Maybe it was the way in which Katie had shared her thoughts and her story in the book or the fact I'd just started a whole new year of endless possibilities – with cancer it would be exactly three in February – but I couldn't help but think it was time to show people that it was possible to live with this disease. Sure, lots of people manage to live with it, and yes, I hadn't even surpassed the three-year typical survival threshold that would make my story remarkable. But surely everything I'd done so far with CoppaFeel! and everything I still wanted to achieve was extraordinary and worth showing others? By 'showing' I meant a documentary. I didn't think I'd have the words yet for a book – I decided more time and experience would help with that – but visually I could tell my story well.

Perhaps a documentary would help us gather even more attention to help us reach our goals? The most recent being: get cancer on the school curriculum. Admittedly an ambitious one, but to us not at all impossible.

Maren and I had become a double act of boob chat, giving talks up and down the country to anything and anyone from big businesses to a SCARY AS HELL TEDx Talk to schools. For almost two years we had been going into schools giving talks to sixth formers and, sometimes, younger kids about why checking their boobs was a really good and very important thing to start doing. Maren's strength to talk about my story and our need to ensure it didn't happen to anyone else sometimes really blew me away. I asked her about it recently; I wanted to know how she really felt about having to share and reshare one of the shittest things that's happened to her. She told me: 'It became a script, to be honest. I was pragmatic when I needed to be. You were well, so that helped. I could hardly start crying to a group of kids, could I? What kind of message would that send? To be honest, I didn't give it that much thought.' I told you she's a keeper!

It was clear from sharing my story so publicly that I was very much not the only one who'd been diagnosed at an early age who needed to make sure others knew. Maren and I couldn't be in every school while also trying to lead an organisation, and so we recruited the Boobettes, a group of badass women who would share their own stories of breast cancer, whether it was a diagnosis or even a scare – a story of someone who found something, had it investigated and was reassured it was nothing is also just as important and powerful. We then even extended it to people who had a strong link to the disease, such as losing mums or sisters to it. The Boobettes swiftly became an army, a family and a force for good; they showed that there are humans behind this insidious disease. What I noticed in them all was something I found in myself too: a need not to dwell, but to focus on something really positive and good whilst also portraying our depth of relief to still be alive. They were turning pain into collective power. I was so proud that we could offer them that. It became one of the most addictive feelings, in fact. Giving someone an opportunity to be a good person made my insides glow.

I couldn't help but start to think that CoppaFeel! shouldn't have to be the ones doing talks in schools about breast cancer. Just as Mar and I couldn't be in every school, we couldn't ensure a Boobette got to every school, at least not very quickly. The enthusiasm from teachers to have us give these sessions made us feel that there was a greater need, one that wasn't met by the curriculum itself. Not just breast cancer but cancer as a whole should be something that is given protected time during a child's life at school. It shouldn't be something that a teacher may or may not take upon themselves to teach in PSHE (personal, social, health and economic education, a doss lesson if you were in my school. I recall being taught how to put a condom on a banana by the head of humanities, who was always covered in dog hairs) if they think it's important enough.

There was no getting around the fact that every single kid in every single school was at some point going to have to deal with cancer, whether that would be their own diagnosis or witnessing someone in their life go through it. It wasn't enough to expect them to learn about it when they were older; it needed to be something they learned about from a young age, ideally before fear of the disease kicks in and, incidentally, when they are adopting new habits anyway. Add to that the fact that almost half of all cancers are preventable with better lifestyle choices.

I'd already been invited to be an 'expert' at a meeting for a new London cancer strategy, led by the then Mayor of London (I mean, I scoffed at the word 'expert', but stepped up to the challenge). They needed patient groups, charities, cancer specialists and more clever people to help them work up a plan of action for cancer awareness in the city and *man* was I more than happy to help. But more than that, I was particularly keen to meet someone whose title jumped off the attendance list I'd been sent ahead of the meeting: a 'human behaviour expert' named Claire McDonald. I made a beeline for her at the meeting, and I decided then and there that she would be my new best friend. And I'm happy to say she still is my friend now and also a trustee of CoppaFeel!

Back then I quizzed her all day long about how we could get young people to *actually* check their boobs, not just once, but for life, and I got her to introduce me to anyone useful for making cancer statutory on the school curriculum. She filled my head full of really fucking cool human behaviour-change examples and I was *hooked*. She joined our mission and together we produced Coppa-Feel!'s Rethink Cancer campaign. Its aim: to make cancer-awareness education in schools a statutory requirement to teach as part of the PSHE curriculum. We wanted:

- All student teachers to be trained how to teach young people how to look after and manage their health.
- All secondary-school students to have protected time in the school curriculum to learn how to look after and manage their health.
- For there to be a creative approach to teaching cancer awareness and healthy behaviours that have impact and tangible benefits.

Sounds cool, huh? Of course I didn't know how we'd eventually convince the right people to make this happen but, undeterred, and with Claire's brilliant brain and wonderful support, I knew we could at best make it happen and at worst get lots of 'bugger off's.

*

A documentary would be another way to reach more people. Now that I'd had the idea, I didn't even wait to get home from holiday to get the wheels in motion. At that stage in my life there was no such thing as 'out of office' – I'd be on emails at any time of the day, on any day of the week, anywhere, even on a campsite on the other side of the world. So there and then I shot an email off to Laura from our PR agency to see if she had any contacts in the TV-production world. It was probably the middle of the night at home but that didn't necessarily mean she wouldn't get back to me straight away – she was always on her phone, and in work mode, possibly more than me.

'I think I know someone,' came her reply.

Back home Maren and I met with a young producer called Neil from October Films. He seemed pretty guarded during the chat; it was only in his follow-up email that he gave any signs that we may be on to something. During the actual chat he seemed reserved but also maybe thoughtful. That was fine; I didn't need anyone blowing smoke up my arse or making any false promises. Just a few short weeks later Neil and I met up to film snippets of my life for a teaser film – a 'sizzle', as he called it. Hopefully it would be enough to get the big dogs at the BBC or Channel 4 or even 5 interested. Just to have the faith of Neil and Matt (his boss) was exciting enough already – surely they would know what gets successfully commissioned these days?

*

Then one day I had a headache. It wasn't like all my other headaches, the ones that had plagued me since I was a kid: this felt different.

11 May 2012

Hi Dr Hope,

Hope you're well.
  I just wondered what you would make of a chronic headache I've had since yesterday morning. I suffer from migraines anyway, but this feels very different. The pain starts at my forehead and goes to the top of my head. I had to stay in bed all day with it yesterday as it made me vomit three times. Painkillers aren't really working and I am taking metoclopramide for the nausea.
  It's unusual for me to be out of action like this, so I thought it might need investigating.
  What do you think?

Kris

He ordered a scan. I had the scan. Then I waited. I have found that waiting bit the most excruciating of all because I know that somewhere, someone – even if it's just the clever imaging machine or the radiographer who

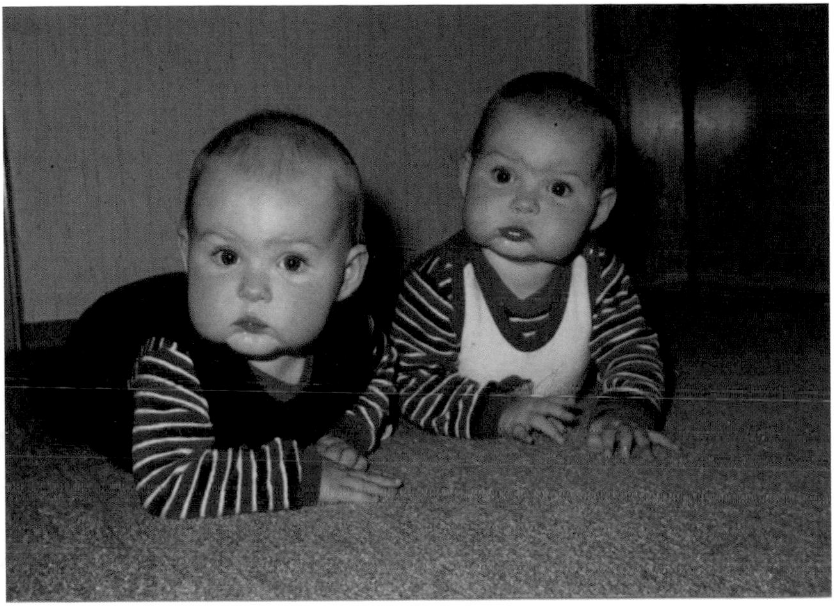

I can confirm we have not grown into our cheeks yet.
Kris *(left)* and Maren, 1985.

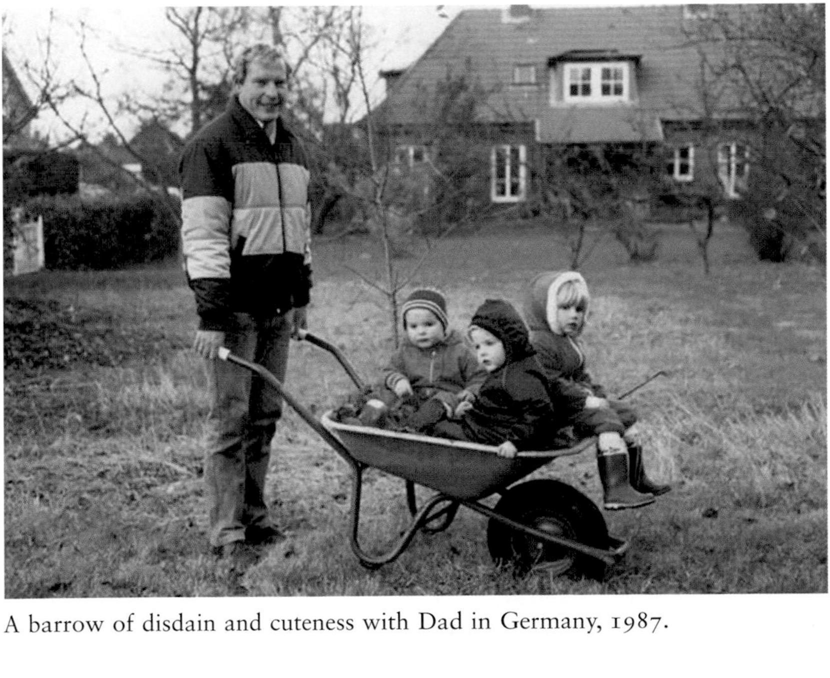

A barrow of disdain and cuteness with Dad in Germany, 1987.

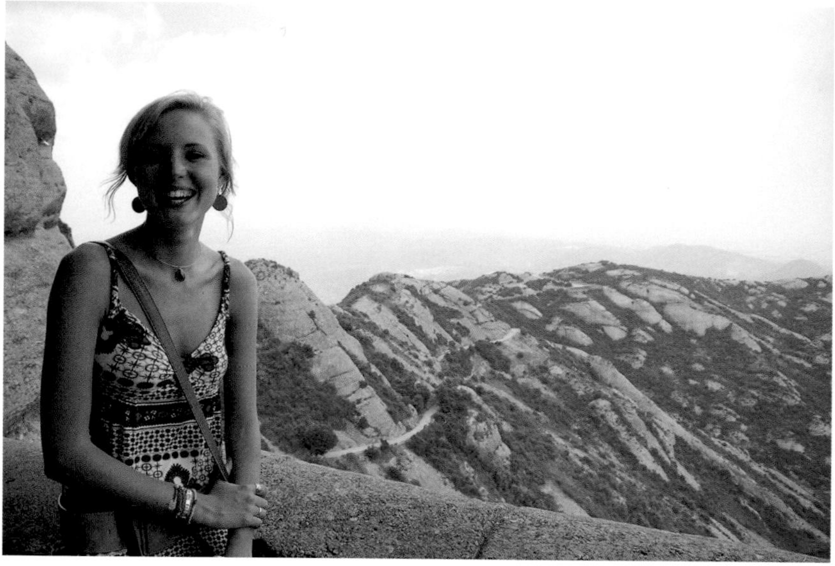

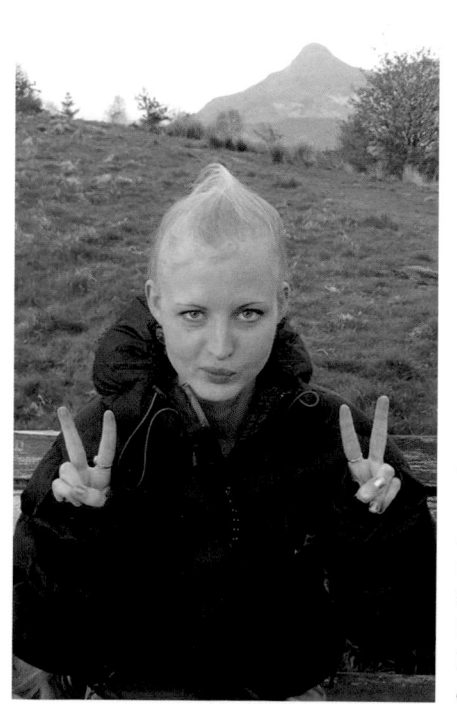

Top: In Barcelona, days before my first trip to the GP in 2008.

Left: An evening sitting by the loch in Glencoe, Scotland, with Niall, brushing all my hair out. I had done the first two cycles of chemo, 2009.

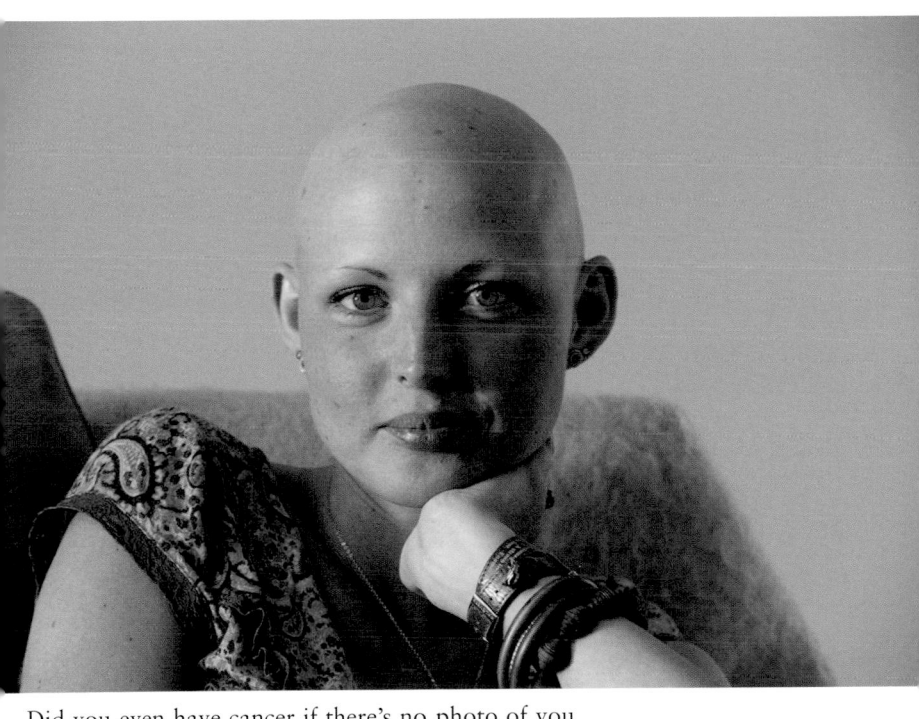

Did you even have cancer if there's no photo of you
receiving chemo with no hair?

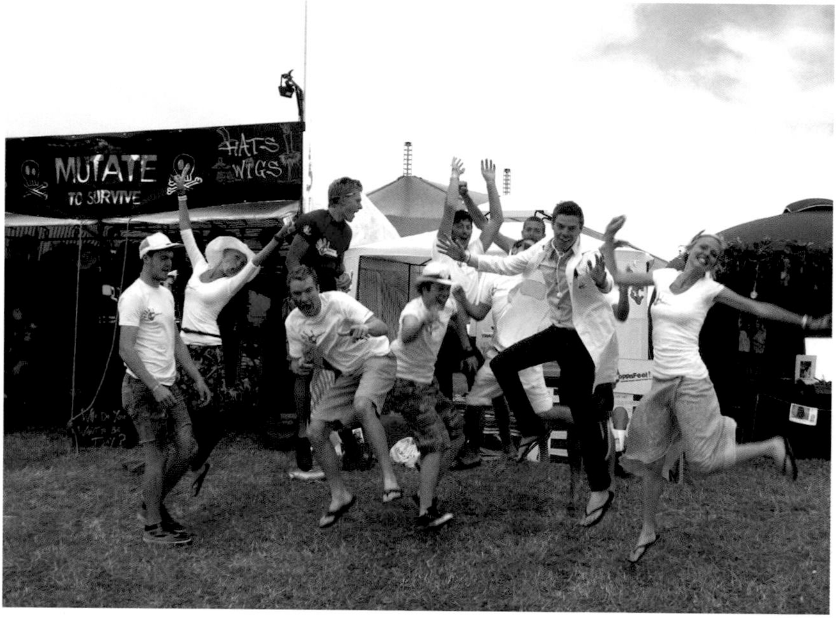

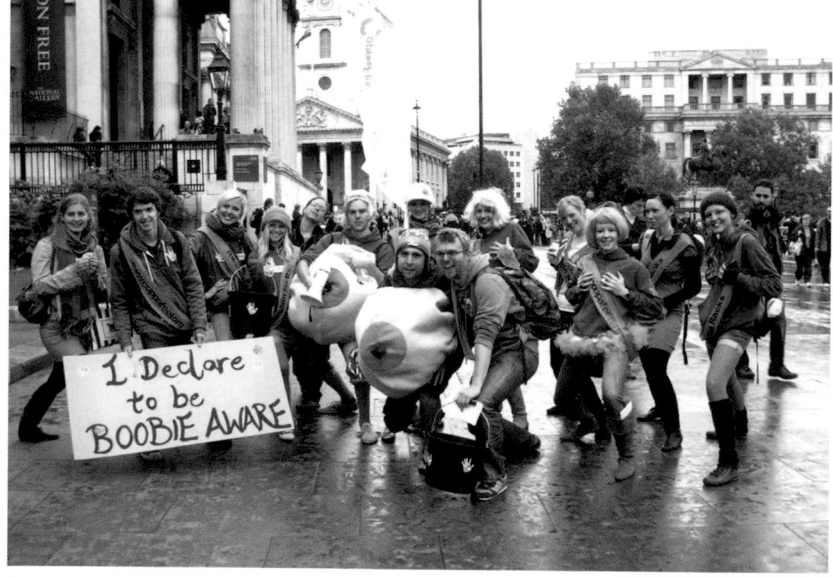

Our very first outing as CoppaFeel!, Beach Break Live, 2009. A crappy gazebo, some stickers, some lads and a red bucket to collect money in.

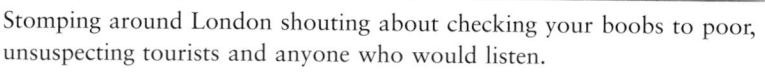

Stomping around London shouting about checking your boobs to poor, unsuspecting tourists and anyone who would listen.

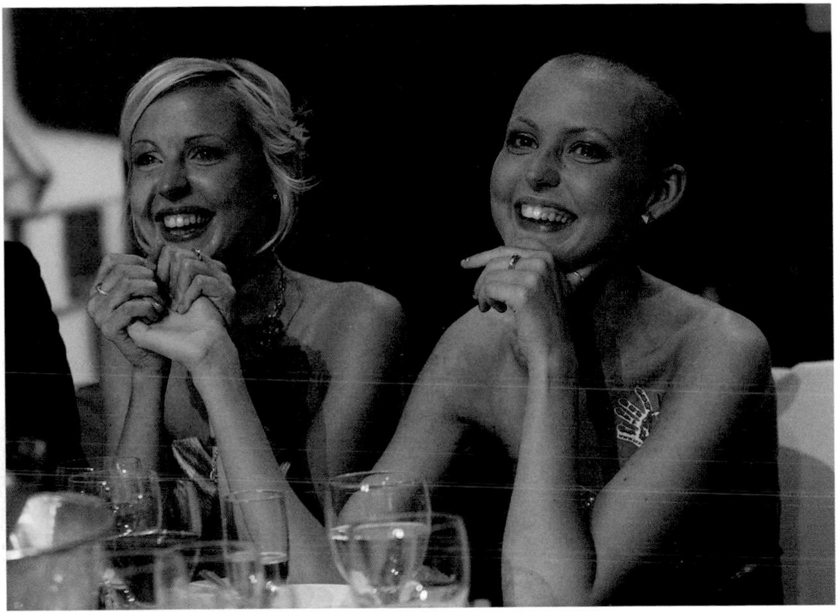

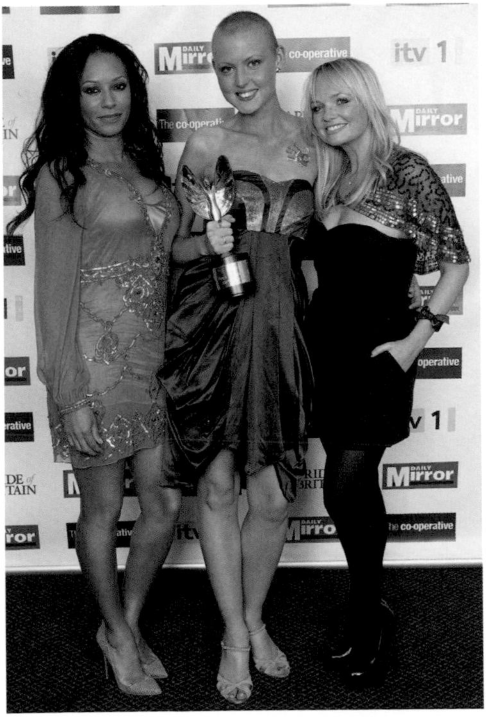

Top: Happy tears at the Pride of Britain Awards.

Left: Awkwardly smiling and playing it cool backstage after receiving my Pride of Britain award from Spice Girls Mel B and Emma Bunton in 2009.

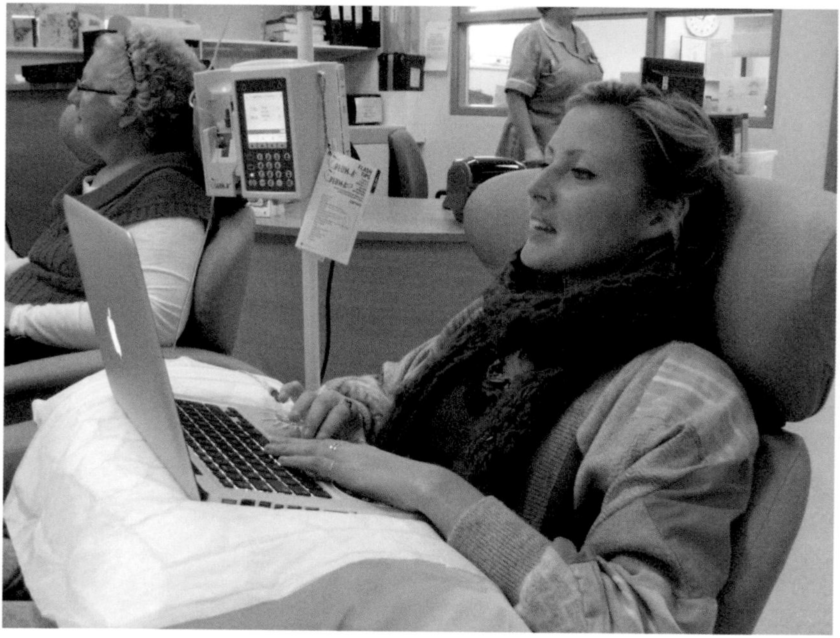

Time spent getting treatment in hospital rarely meant downtime.

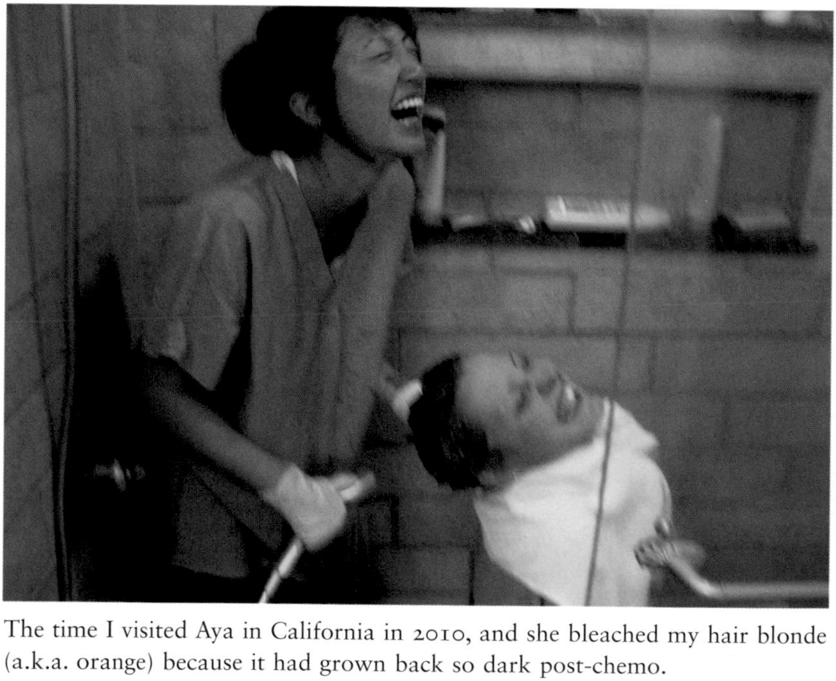

The time I visited Aya in California in 2010, and she bleached my hair blonde (a.k.a. orange) because it had grown back so dark post-chemo.

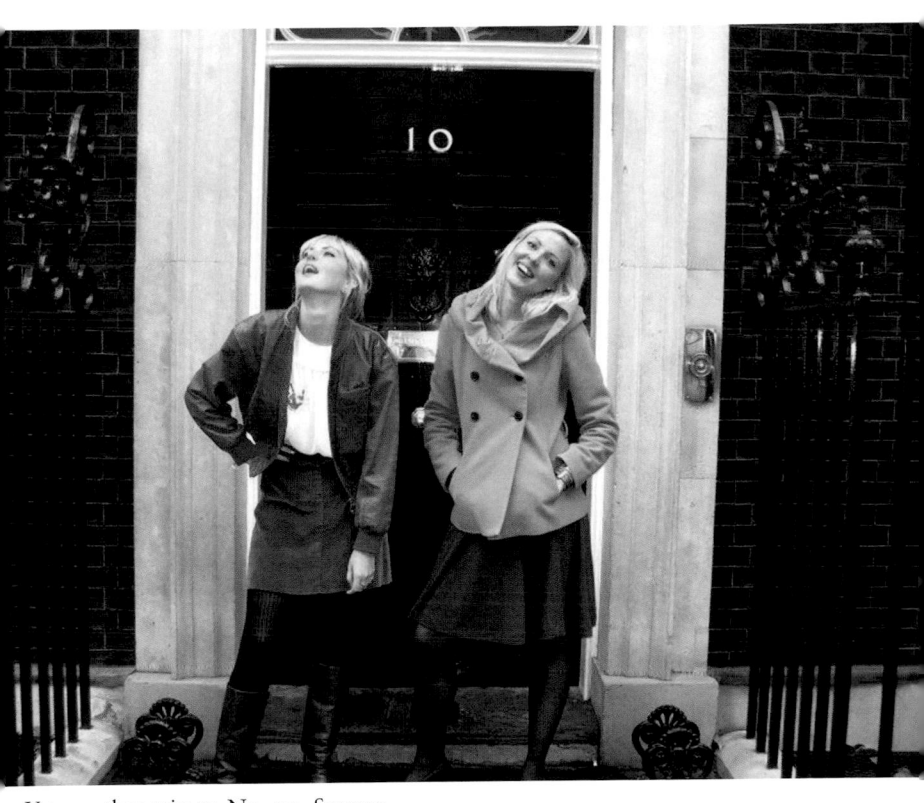

Yet another trip to No. 10. Snooze.

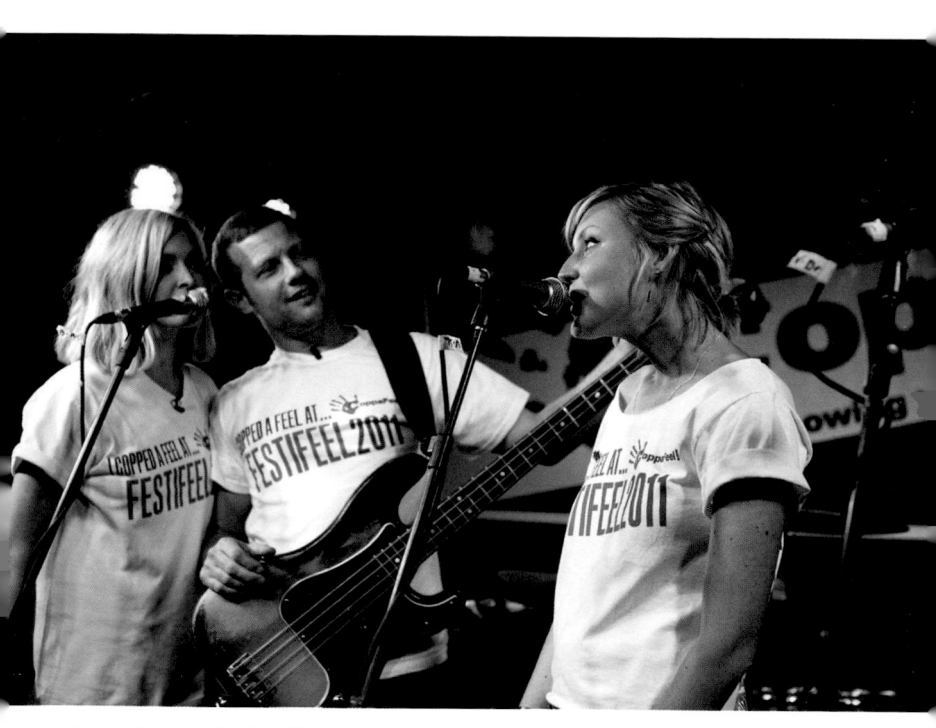

Introducing the headline act at our second
Festifeel in 2011, with our amazing patrons
Fearne Cotton and Dermot O'Leary.

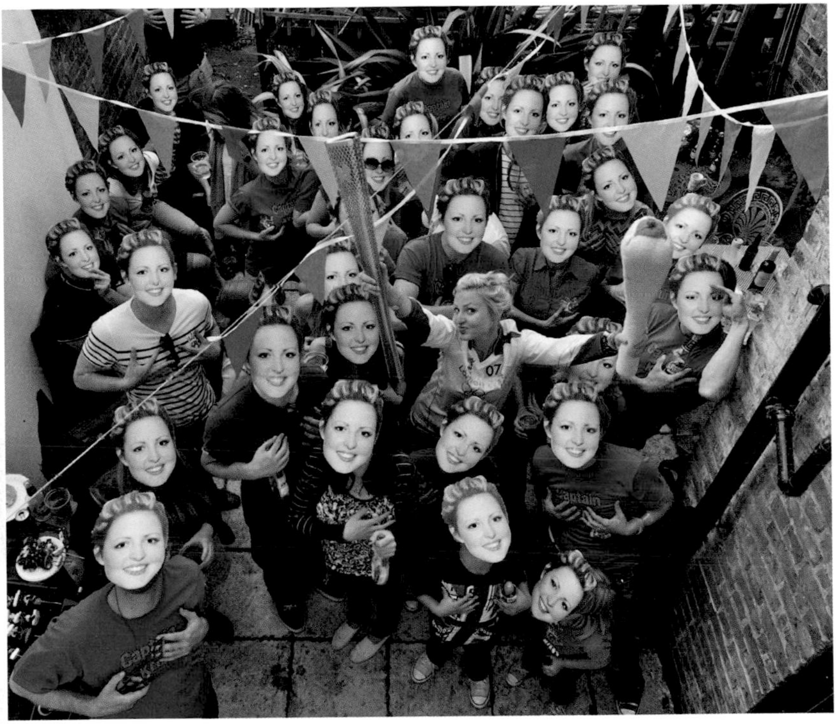

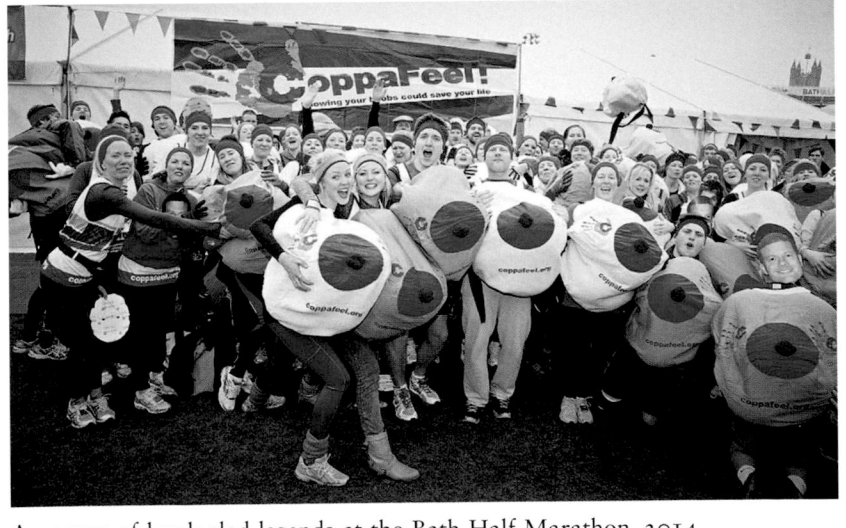

A creepy day: surrounded by all my favourite people who were wearing my face after I ran in the torch relay for the London Olympics 2012.

An ocean of boob-clad legends at the Bath Half Marathon, 2014.

Image courtesy of Danny North

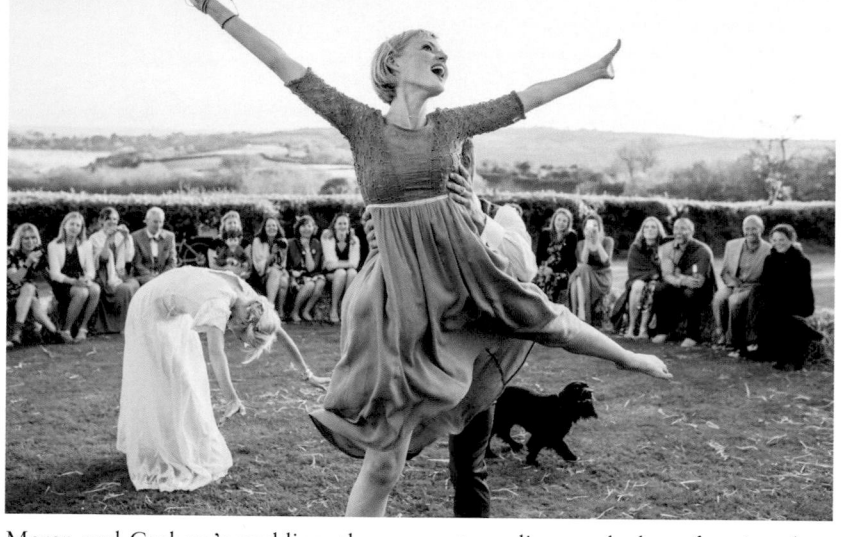

Maren and Graham's wedding: the moment our lives peaked, performing the dance from *Romy and Michele's High School Reunion*.

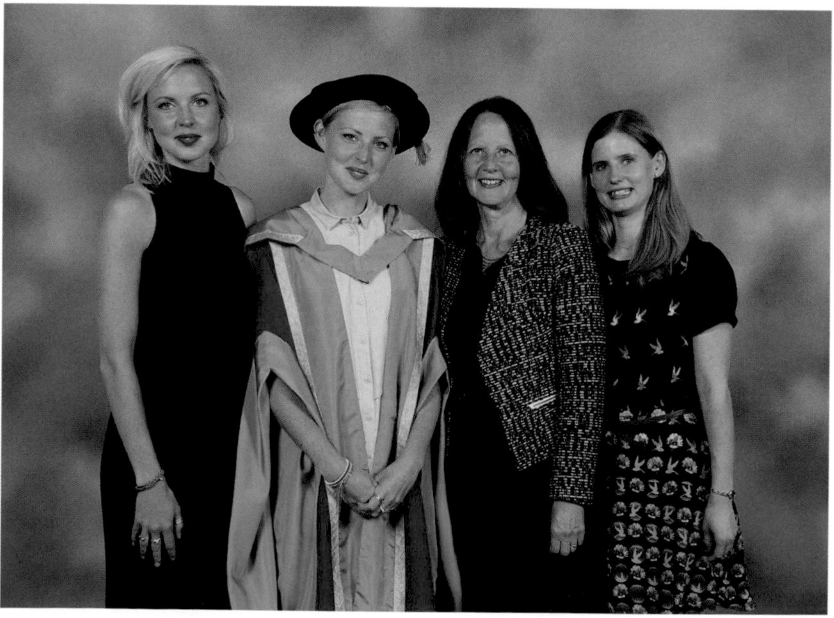

Wearing a colourful cape and a floppy hat with Maren, Mum and Maike at my honorary doctorate graduation at Nottingham Trent University, 2015.

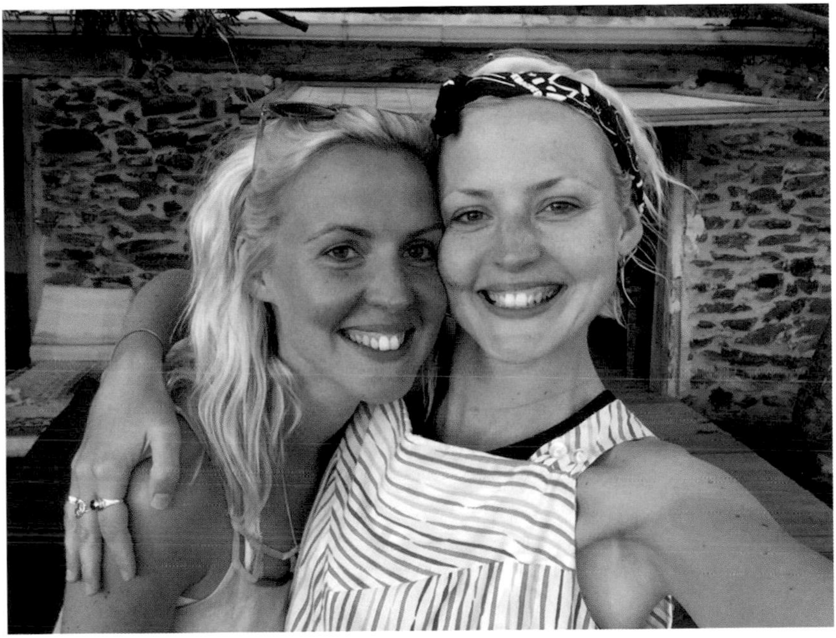

Alive to do those things: go to Italy with Maren, 2016.

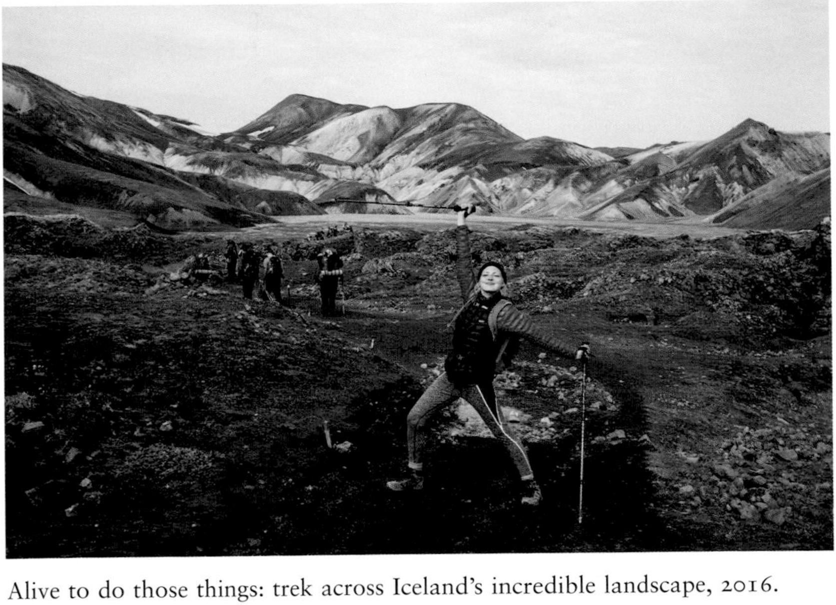

Alive to do those things: trek across Iceland's incredible landscape, 2016.

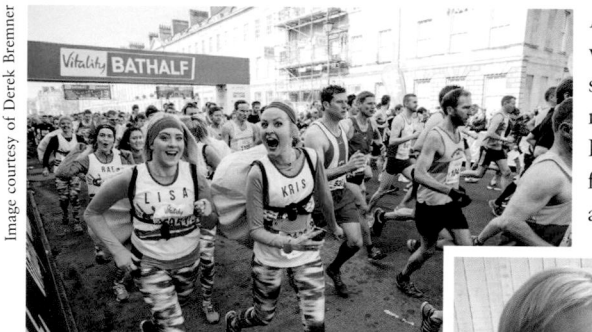

Image courtesy of Derek Bremner

Left: I do not know who this is but she somehow ran a half marathon with her pal Lisa, shortly after finding out she had another brain tumour.

Right: With Jenny on her wedding day: seven years after she emailed me to say she had been diagnosed with breast cancer aged twenty-six, and wouldn't have gone back to the GP if it hadn't been for me sharing my own story.

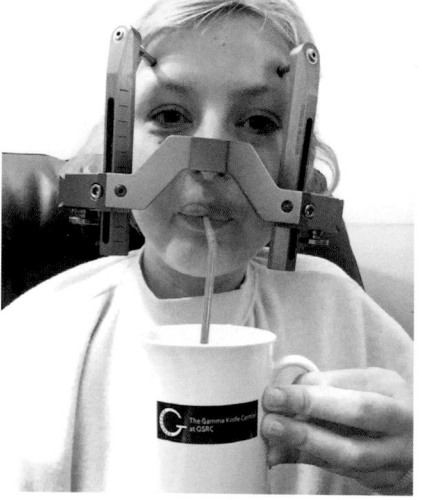

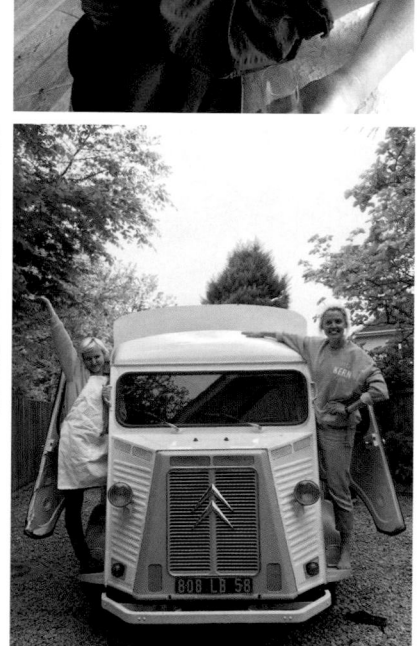

Above: A contraption screwed to my head so I would lie as still as possible for one of many brain tumour zapping gamma knife treatments at Queen Square, London, in 2018.

Right: Our first outing with Beyoncé, the cake and coffee truck, 2017.

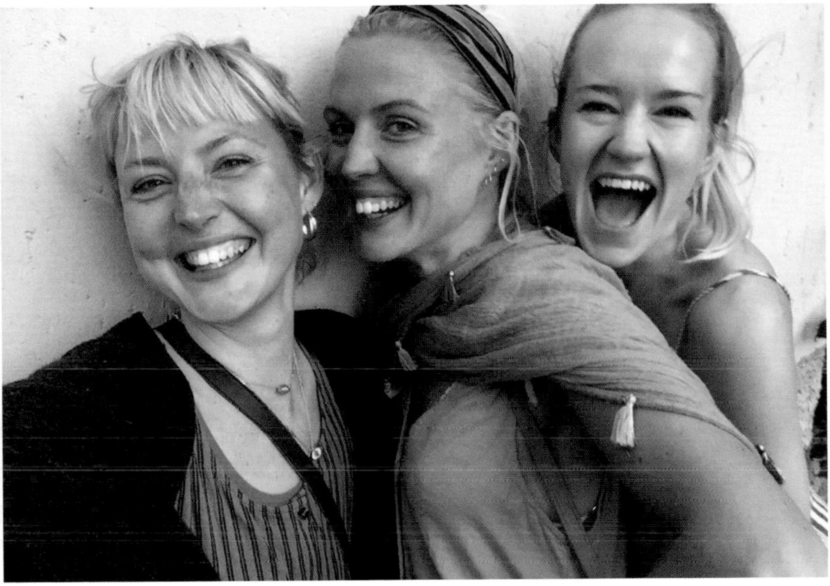

A rare moment of pure happiness with Maren and Stacey on holiday in Italy during one of the toughest years of my life, 2018.

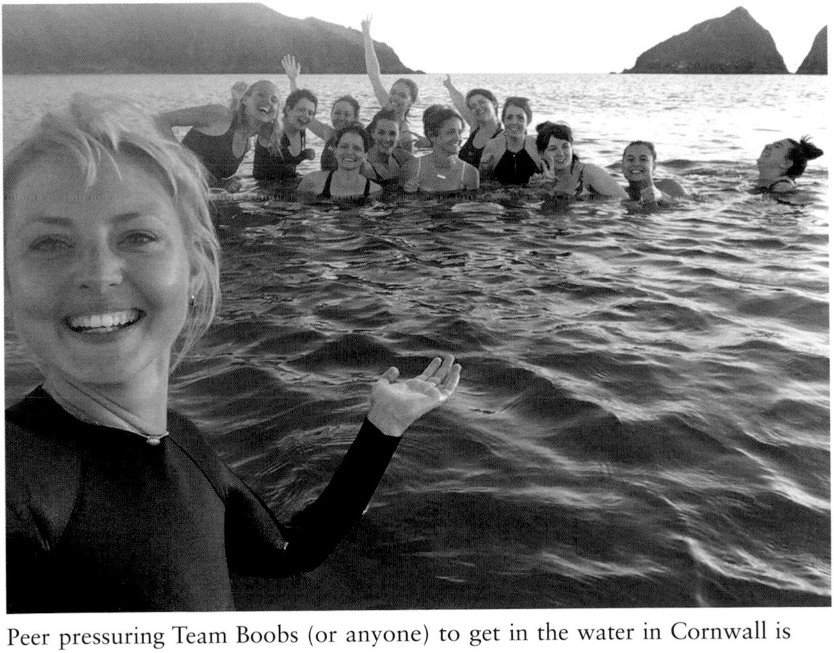

Peer pressuring Team Boobs (or anyone) to get in the water in Cornwall is one of my favourite pastimes.

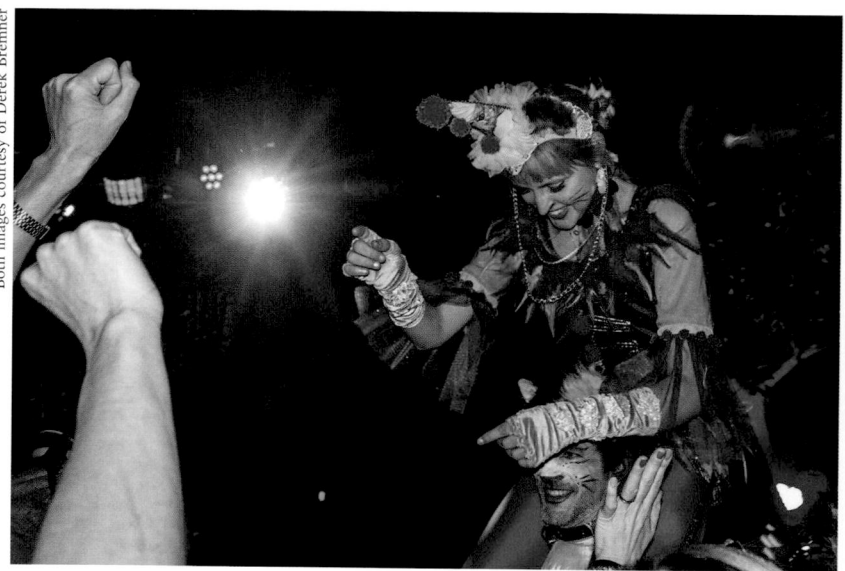

A very low-key cat-themed party at the Eden Project in Cornwall, to celebrate ten years of not dying of cancer, 2019.

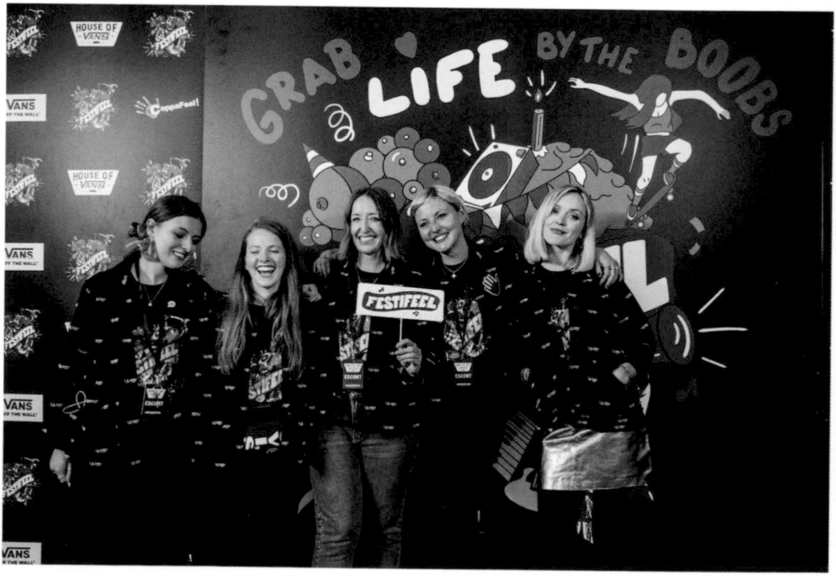

Women that keep the world spinning: my Festifeel crew, 2019.

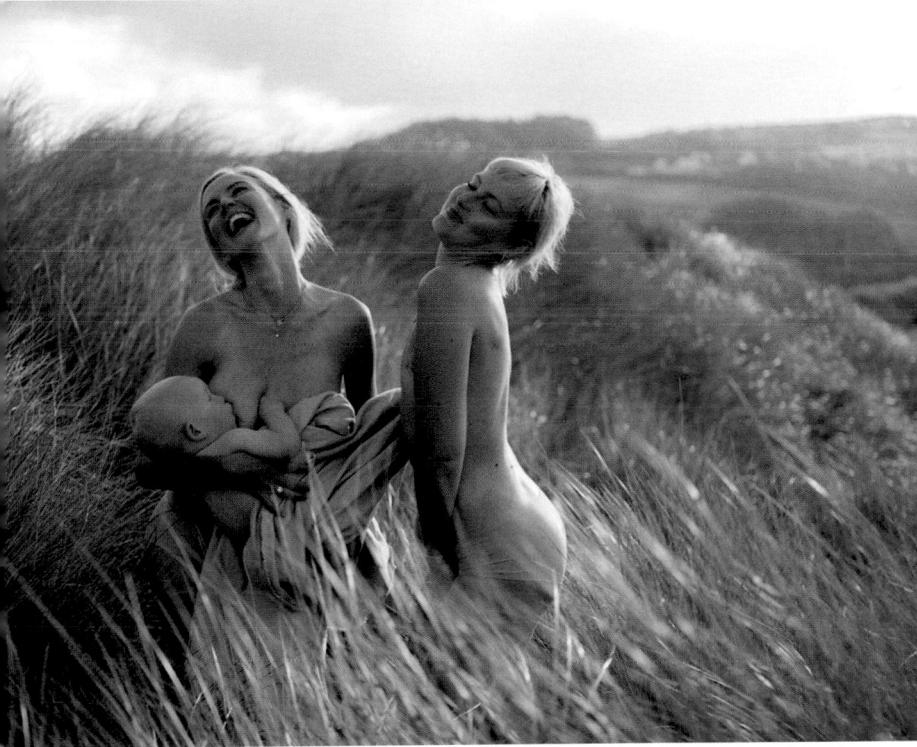

Just a pretty average morning in the Cornish dunes, post-second mastectomy, with Maren and Herbie, 2020. All jokes aside, it's a pretty poignant photo: boobs for sustaining life, and no boobs for sustaining life.

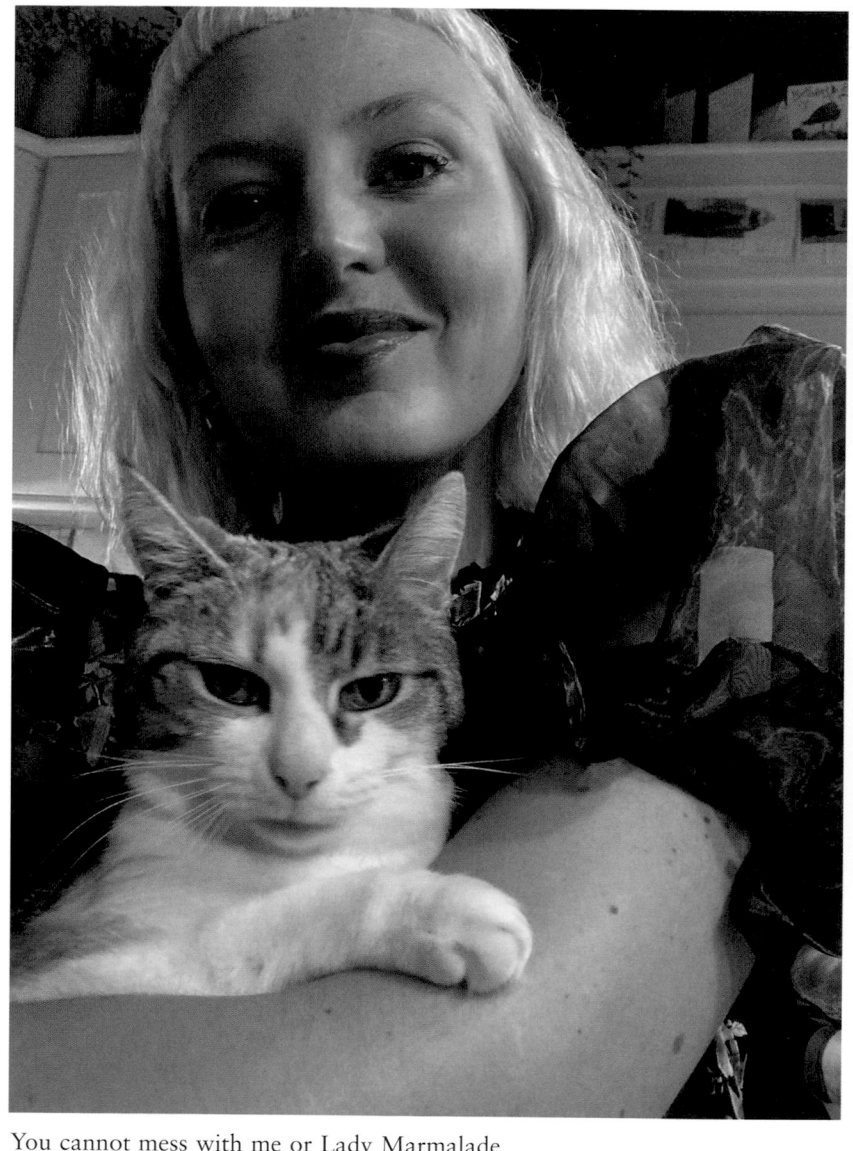

You cannot mess with me or Lady Marmalade
(but mostly Lady Marmalade).

might be looking at the images and writing up a report about what they can see – knows something that I don't. And it's inevitable that I will find out whatever it is he or she now knows. I've often considered if there could be value in never knowing. Alas, there isn't. During the days before scan results I'm not really myself. I can hold a conversation, but I don't really feel like I'm in my body. I'm on high alert, which means I can't be fully present. I can't be in that moment because I'm too worried about the next moment. I sometimes go for a walk. Have a bath. Read and escape to someone else's life for a bit (if you're doing that now, hi! I hope my shit makes your shit more doable).

I hadn't heard from Dr Hope and I couldn't wait for my next appointment, so I sent him a quick email with, 'I guess no news is good news?'

'I will call you shortly,' came his reply. And the call came. And with it the news every inch of my mind was dreading, and my stomach was seemingly readying itself for. I did indeed have a brain tumour (there are four places breast cancer *really, really* loves to go more than others: liver, bones, lungs and brain. Three out of four now achieved. But not quite at the bingo call yet). A tiny one. Two millimetres. I was at home when I took that call. Shortly after, I paced up and down the living room trying to regain some kind of normal breathing pattern and heart rate. I shared the news with Mum, Maike and Maren, but also with my camera.

'Twenty-ninth of May 2012. The day that I found out I have a brain tumour,' I announced down the barrel of my SLR lens. The news surely couldn't have sunk in by that point, not really, but I wanted to ensure whenever I did my camera diaries I was being as up to date and authentic as possible. I'd only be making this documentary once and I was hell-bent on making it real. Just when I dared to think that I was doing quite well and cancer wasn't wrecking my party quite so much – that it was tamed to just being the drunken friend slumped in the corner, rather than the guy who is setting his farts on fire and vomming everywhere, if you get me – BAM, I got that smackdown. It's not the news that hurts, it's the not knowing what to do next. I'm better with a plan of action. The standing at the crossroads bit is the bit I fear.

What followed was some radiotherapy, called stereo-tactic radiotherapy, to the tiny, almost microscopic brain lesion they had found. It involved getting a very tight mask fitted to keep my head super still while beams blasted the tumour from lots of different angles, all meeting at the cancer. Being so targeted meant that the tumour received a high dose of radiation and the tissues around it received a much lower dose, ensuring very few side effects and less long-term damage to my precious brain. Although having cancer in my brain was terrifying – I mean, it had for so long been one of my rainiest-day scenarios – the treatment was by far one of the easiest I'd had, especially when compared to the likes of, I dunno, the spinal drilling during the vertebroplasty. I would just need to hope that this was a little blip, that the cancer wouldn't decide to pop up anywhere new.

Thankfully Dr Hope didn't want to drastically change my systemic treatment. He obviously wasn't too happy that my current treatment wasn't halting further spread, but it still didn't prove that it was rampant, out-of-control spread. And so, once the stereotactic radiotherapy was done, I continued on my hormone treatment.

'We got the green light from BBC Three,' came the excited words from Neil. By the summer we had bagged ourselves a BBC Three commission. I had no reference to whether that was lucky, unusual or normal, but I soon learned that first-time commissions, with as random a story as mine (not fitting within a 'theme' they were programming, that is), wasn't typical at all.

Almost a year of filming ensued. What started off as a film to showcase our work and plea to get cancer on the curriculum also turned into therapy for me. I would share my innermost, squirrelled-away thoughts and feelings and worries with Neil. Whether it was just Neil's skill at squeezing it all out of me or because I needed a camera to help me find my voice sometimes, either way it all helped to shape a film that was a true representation of me, of a life with cancer at that time. True were the words I spoke about cancer and the fear and frustration surrounding my life, and true were the words I spoke of the pain I was feeling breaking up with Catface. I mean, SURE the best time to break up with someone is when you're making a TV documentary, right?

When Catface and I first got together, what I loved most about him was that he helped me to forget I had cancer. It felt like he didn't mind that we might not have a future together, that the present was all that mattered. Thinking back now, he never said those words, but that's what I told myself – after all, I was well versed in telling myself how a relationship was going even if it was far from the truth. I'd thought that cancer would mean that no one would want to be with me, but he seemed able to treat our relationship as any other perfectly normal relationship. Except, of course, it wasn't.

As time went on – and I endured more and more treatments – I started to resent that he wouldn't acknowledge my illness and the reality of my condition. I'd taken his ability not to be shaken or shocked by anything as a sign of strength, but more and more it felt like nonchalance and ignorance – all the ances, in fact. Most of the time he wouldn't come with me to the hospital for my routine appointments, or to tests or even results; always afraid to,

God forbid, ask for a day off. And yeah, I know there was a lot of them. But over time it served as a way to make me think it wasn't a big deal, and if it wasn't a big deal then I mustn't be scared. I wasn't allowed to be scared.

The truth was, some days I did need to offload, to tell him how petrified I was and cry until I fell asleep. I didn't need him to move me out of my grief or pain; he could have let me sit with it. Instead of allowing me to feel what I needed to feel, he felt he needed to solve a problem. I didn't need him to have the answers; I just needed him to distract me and make me feel like my world wasn't caving in. I didn't want a fuss but I did need a hand-squeeze from time to time, and without having to ask. I needed to put coping and positivity and a brave face to one side for a minute and let it the fuck out.

I realised things were really bad with him and just the weight of absolutely everything when I couldn't stop crying for three days. I wished I could put it down to hormones, but I no longer had something to blame my mood swings on, since I was post-menopausal (although, having said that, I do think, periods or no periods, we all have a deep-set natural cycle no matter what, but more on that another day, perhaps). I allowed myself three whole days to wallow in this deep, all-consuming, guttural sadness before deciding there was something bigger at play and something I needed help with. But up until then I just allowed myself to feel whatever I needed to feel without any shame or regret. I was sad, FFS. I needed everyone else around me to say, *Man, your life is well shit, isn't it?* Of course they didn't, and in reality my life was far, FAR from shit, but I needed to acknowledge the hard stuff. Not coping is not a sign of weakness.

We'd moved in together within a year of meeting and with that came a sort of stale routine that irritated me. I never wanted to have to remind anyone that I had an illness that was constantly reminding me of my mortality, but sometimes I just couldn't help it – I was desperate to be heard. It's a pretty sorry state of affairs if you find yourself reminding someone you're dying to get them to show a little interest in doing something nice together, isn't it?

Was the ultimate demise of our relationship all his fault? Nope. The non-existent gap between me trying to get over my past relationships and diving head first into another without even allowing any time to process the cancer thing became very apparent too, and it was nobody's fault but my own. I hadn't unlearned my self-loathing yet. Sure Catface never, ever made me feel like I was worthless, and I knew that when he said he loved me, he really meant it – he wasn't one to express his emotions much – but my past relationships had left me riddled with doubt and uncertainty. I thought the very fact that I managed to be in a relationship despite me, on paper, being far from a catch, would be enough to boost my confidence again, but I was so wrong. I needed constant reassurance.

I questioned myself and my behaviour all the time in fear of being or becoming the 'psycho' girlfriend. I was petrified that I wasn't good enough, and who could blame me? I hadn't yet regained the self-value that had been stripped away from me. Winning the Pride of Britain award, being the boss of my own charity, seeing my resolve in the face of deadly adversity, in short, becoming the CEO of my own life, had built up my sense of self, but it still wasn't enough to bolster my assurance in a relationship. In truth, Catface could have been the Noah character played by Ryan Gosling in *The Notebook* (my ultimate benchmark for a perfect man) and I would have probably still been just as insecure and fearful of doom.

Cancer throws a magnifying lens on just about every aspect of your life, making you question the worth and value of everything. This can sometimes be really helpful if you're deliberating about whether, for example, to clean the house or sack it off and have a day out with people you love (OK yeah, a.k.a. an excuse to be lazy). Perhaps a better example is that it helps you see what truly matters – whether that's the people you choose to continue being friends with and have in your life, how you wish to spend your days and whether you should blow a few hundred quid on a treehouse holiday (the answer is always YES). The downside is the enormous pressure and hold it has on every decision. The emphasis on perfection in my post-diagnosis relationship became suffocating and all-consuming. Too often I'd waste time deliberating whether it was really all worth my time and effort when all I should have done was go with the flow like every other healthy human might. Ironically, I tried too hard to be happy, to the detriment of my own happiness.

I've been more terrified of not being loved when I've been in a relationship than when I've not been. I could never get comfortable knowing that Catface was my life partner but I was more than likely not his. That imbalance of importance made my insecurities skyrocket. A relationship with cancer is loaded and heavy – how could it not be? There is no freedom to 'see where it might go'; there is only ever the thought that it may end very tragically and yes, before you say it, I know this could very much be the case for any couple *ever*, but for us it was way more, ya know, *real*. I put more pressure on it to be perfect because nothing less would do. In other words, you're exhausted before you even have to deal with the fact he left the toilet seat up.

Not only is the being in love bit hard work, but the breaking-up bit is even worse. I spent a long time being sad about the fact I may have wasted four precious years of my allocated 'still alive' time – this wasn't just general bog-standard heartbreak. At the risk of sounding irreparably tragic, I've done more crying over breaking up with a boy than over cancer and my dad's death combined. I berated myself for not exiting sooner or knowing better. Break-ups are hard enough without naughty cancer cells roaming your body, and I can tell you that no amount of Cadbury's Dairy Milk helps the regret you feel about having been in a relationship that now seems meaningless when time is so tight. Except, of course, that it wasn't at all meaningless, but it's taken seven years to reach that conclusion. I now don't regret a single decision. A single plea. My desperation. The many tears. You do, after all, have to kiss a few frogs, as my nanna rightly said.

You see, the fact is this: cancer doesn't in any way make you less blinded by love, however much you think you might be more in control of your thoughts and feelings and priorities. With or without cancer, *love is still a bitch*. I can't imagine how different those years might have been had I not chosen to be with him – certainly we would have had a way shittier website – but really there is no need to even think about that.

I had never 'done' cancer without him. (Well, except the first four months, but that's when I was still telling my ex to fuck off/was in shock that I had breast cancer.) For those first four years of cancer I had someone I lay next to in bed that I could curl tightly up to when everything seemed too heavy. He was there during some of the hardest, ickiest days of my life and ridiculous ones too – like that time I overdosed on morphine from a fentanyl patch and threw up so much I had to go to A & E and subsequently hallucinated that Fireman Sam was coming through the ceiling of the hospital as the anti-emetics were kicking in. Being with me was a real barrel of laughs. We'd experienced all the tricky, sticky, magical edges of life together.

Once I even saw him cry (with pride or love or overwhelming fondness – at least, that's what I told myself) as I carried the Olympic torch through the streets of East London. I mean, I was crying too. Lining the streets were all my most precious people wearing masks of my face and T-shirts saying 'Boob Chief Kris' and, most bizarrely of all, complete strangers were thrusting their babies and small children into my arms for photos. I felt like Princess Diana. We adopted a cat called Wilhelm together (who I got to keep in the divorce); he rinsed my sick bucket; he calmed me and reassured me. He didn't always say the right things or do the necessary things, but he tickled my head, cooked me dinner at the end of a long, stressful day and showed me how it felt to be loved unconditionally, warts – or should I say tumours – and all. It's hard to believe, I know, but trust me when I say I believe in love even after my disastrous relationship history. I still hold on to that nugget of belief, I do. I love love.

*

It was in the wake of our break-up that I discovered hospice care. Yup, I know what you're thinking because I thought it too: *That's where you go to die.* But I was wrong and so are you. Hospice care and palliative care are focused on making you live better, not die sooner. Perhaps it should be called 'help you live' care. I obviously never got told this by my medical team: this was once again something I had to figure out myself. Turns out that palliative care can even make you live longer! Researchers at US university Tulane examined the impact of outpatient palliative care on over 2,000 advanced cancer patients' survival and quality of life. Fifty-six per cent of patients who were randomised to receive outpatient palliative care were alive after one year as opposed to 42 per cent who received typical care. That split doesn't sound that significant, but in terms of time left on this planet, it gave palliative care patients more than four months longer than their counterparts who did not receive palliative care.

I did some digging to find somewhere that might offer reflexology to cancer patients – bloody lovely foot-massage treatment – and soon realised the plethora of places where I could access this. Oh London, I love you. The moment I stepped through the doors at Marie Curie in Hampstead was the day my life got easier, lighter even. You get allocated a consultant, like a proper doctor, who deals with the stuff your oncologist will never bring up, such as your mental stability. Mine also asked me what was *right*, not always what was wrong.

Dr Faye Gishen, my assigned consultant, who would prove to be a lifeline on more than one occasion, asked me whether I'd ever tried antidepressants. It was the last thing I thought she'd suggest. For four years I'd only ever dealt with doctors who cared for the cancer, and the cancer only. Never had someone asked me about my mental health, how I was coping and whether I needed help. And boy did I need help. She prescribed me a super-low dose of citalopram to 'take the edge off', as not only was I now dealing with the Catface break-up but my landlord was selling my home and *ugh*, it all felt too much. She suggested I take it until I felt I could deal with life again. I had been so anti antidepressants, but they helped me then and still help me today. Suffer less, live more.

And that wasn't the only thing she suggested. She asked me how much I exercised. At this point I'd lost all confidence in 'working out'. My body had been through so much, and when I had asked my oncologist just six months after my diagnosis if I could run a half-marathon alongside all my friends in support of CoppaFeel! (admittedly that was a silly suggestion) he advised against it. I didn't feel like I belonged in a gym: that was for healthy people. There had been a phase in my life where I was obsessed with exercising, but that wasn't me any more.

On doing a quick leg-strength test, Dr Gishen told me I needed to exercise, as it wouldn't just help my body stay strong but help me mentally too. And she was so right. I joined the local council gym and I started to see just how powerful movement would be for helping me believe I was healthy and for thinking happier and healthier thoughts in general.

And all the while this was happening, filming for the documentary was going on. When I wasn't talking to hospice staff, I was talking to Neil on camera. He had the power to make me cry in just about any public space. Clissold Park has seen and felt a lot of my tears. When I wasn't talking to him, I was walking, or meeting someone like a young girl called Laura in Dorset, who had just been diagnosed with breast cancer, or MPs in Westminster. For the finale of the film we needed a bit of a stunt. We needed to show just how important changing the curriculum was and the lengths I would go to to see it happen, and also, you know, make good telly. One hare-brained idea led to another until we decided we should project the statistic that one in three people get cancer on to the Houses of Parliament. Ultimately it was the people within those walls who had the power to effect real change. I'd seen it done before when Gail Porter's naked body was splashed in bright lights onto the building for *FHM* magazine. This would, hopefully, make better headlines.

Of course, I didn't have a clue how to go about it, and because our commission was from the BBC my production crew couldn't be seen to be organising anything potentially illegal. So it fell on me to organise a projection company (in other words beg them, because believe it or not, stealth companies pulling off stunts like these don't tend to want to be seen in a documentary) and try to find the money to cover the costs. The universe and I (plus our dear friend Harry, who happened to know people who could raise £2,500 overnight to cover the cost of the projection) conspired to make it happen, and one chilly evening in early 2013 Maren and I found ourselves on Waterloo Bridge staring at our capital's Parliament building with a hand-drawn image of our then three party leaders – Ed Miliband, David Cameron and Nick Clegg – with the words '1 in 3* are diagnosed #Rethink Cancer' and, fucking hell, we had never felt more badass. Until, of course, a policeman came plodding along to the sound of helicopters overhead (probably unrelated, but it adds to the suspense, OK?), asking us to stop the projection and filming immediately. Neil secretly kept rolling as I word-vomited my sob story and mission to the policeman, who by the end just simply said, 'Go home.' I think

---

* It is now 1 in 2, FYI.

he'd heard enough or got bored. But we'd done it. We successfully managed to keep the images up for about ten minutes, which is pretty much a record for a stunt like that, especially post 9/11.

It would be a few more weeks of filming and waiting before *Kris: Dying to Live* was eventually scheduled for TV in March 2014, viewed by 500k on the first night, and then by thousands on iPlayer days and months later. It would be another three years until we would finally hear that cancer was being added to a now statutory PSHE curriculum from September 2020, thanks to the collective hassling by us and other equally desperate parties. Collective power at its best.

C-Word, The Movie

Life is never incomplete if it is an honourable one.
At whatever point you leave life, if you leave it in the
right way, it is whole.

Seneca

Nothing about breast cancer online forums or meet-ups
made me want to join them – not helped by the fact that
my breast cancer nurse declared, the day I was diagnosed,
that there was a local group I could join but I'd 'be the
youngest person there'. Thanks but no thanks. But I also
didn't see why you'd want to sit around talking about
breast cancer with people you don't know; to me that
seemed like a waste of precious life. Cancer was a club I
never asked to join, so I never subscribed to the 'sister-
hood' idea – that just because we all have the same
disease, we should all be the best of friends. I have news
for you: it is possible to be a knob before, during, and
even after breast cancer. Shocking as it may seem, cancer

doesn't automatically mean we have anything other than mutant cells in common. If I like you it's because I like *you*, not the fact we both suffer from hot flushes and dry vaginas. (Although the one and only time I did go to a group session, for a pilot conducted by Breast Cancer Care, for young women with secondary breast cancer, they handed out free lube, which would, unbeknownst to my then still averagely moist vajay, come in handy later on. These meetings have their place – I get it.)

But then I met Fran. Someone who also had breast cancer – primary to start with, and treated 'successfully', only for it to spread not long after and become secondary and incurable like mine. Whether it was the knowledge that she had experienced the exact same breathtaking fears about dying as I had that created our kinship (and thus contradicting and negating what I just said above) or whether she was just a really fucking cool chick, I don't know. I am going to go with both.

I met Fran on a magazine shoot. Four of us were done up to the nines in evening dresses and dark, smoky eye make-up, clutching fake cocktails at a bar that reeked of alcohol at eleven in the morning, somewhere in Soho. Each of us had a different type of cancer and right now I don't recall the actual point of the article, and why we all had to look so not like ourselves, but I do know that yet again I saw it as an opportunity to share my story. Fran had me laughing within minutes of us meeting in the lift, where she recognised me from a TV interview, I think.

I was by now quite in the public eye, having done numerous interviews about myself and CoppaFeel!, and people recognised me from the *Pride of Britain Awards* too, months (and actually even now) after transmission. I still wasn't really sure how to handle the attention. I never knew what to say when someone called me 'inspirational'. Cancer is not a badge of honour – let's stamp out that trite narrative. The word 'inspirational' should be reserved for people who have done something or achieved something, not given by virtue of a deadly disease – if so, we should be calling anyone with heart failure inspirational too, shouldn't we? I will now only accept that compliment if you can tell me how I inspired you to *do* something, or *feel* something, or made you check your boobs. Thankfully Fran didn't call me inspirational.

'I've seen you on the telly,' she said, smiling.

'Ah. Yes. Maybe,' I bumbled.

I came to love her no-bullshit approach to being ill. At that point her cancer was still contained and she'd only recently finished treatment for primary breast cancer. We kept in touch via text and email. Even when her breast cancer came back and spread to her lungs, she would often be the voice of reason, the boost and encouragement I would need to get me through yet another scan or wobble. She came with me and held my hand the day I had to have a mask fitted for the radiotherapy to my brain tumour. We'd never dwell or moan or ask why, but sharing our treatment options and asking the questions that both of us shielded from loved ones helped like I never imagined (and yeah, OK, it's probably the kind of comfort you might get at a support group, but we had way more than cancer to talk about!).

There was a day when she'd received bad news – all she seemed to be receiving towards the end – and as I stood in the stairwell at our offices, all I could do was listen to her fears about what to do next. Whether she should try *another* round of chemotherapy, or if, perhaps, enough was enough (in the end she tried *eight*). I can never be sure if I helped her at all in those moments, but I hope I did. I hope that in at least airing stuff she was too frightened to share with the really close people in her life, she could unburden herself a little. Equally, she became that person for me, too. It was towards the end of her life that my respect for her really exploded. She faced it all with such clarity and candour and grace. She blew me away and all I could hope was that I'd have an ounce of her strength when I neared my death. Even days before she died she cared more for telling me that I was far from my own doom than bothering me with hers. 'You're way off this' she wrote (how did she know?). She became my poster girl for how to live, and how to die.

In one of her last ever blog posts she shared the news that the cancer had spread rapidly and extensively throughout her body and there was nothing more she or the hospital would be doing to stop it, and at the end she wrote:

> *I am not afraid of dying. Not any more. Me and death will be just fine because everybody dies; it's what happens. I haven't gone yet. I'm still here. With a sense of humour and a personality and a very clear sense of who I am, which I never had pre-cancer. And that's a gift in itself.*

A sense of who I am is something I strived for because of her.

Part of my research during the early cancer days was reading books by women who seemed to have the cancer thing figured out, which included *Crazy Sexy Cancer Tips* by Kris Carr (it's true, I liked her particularly because we have the same name) and *The C-Word*, Lisa Lynch's extended version of her hilarious blog. When I read it I never imagined we would at some stage – three years later, in fact – be meeting face to face, perched at a picnic table outside my office. Lisa was as funny in real life as she was in the pages of her book. Again, like Fran, I loved her silliness and honesty in the face of all the non-stop cancer shit. We schemed media stuff together. We thought we'd write something like *The Vagina Monologues*, but for boobs, a great idea that never actually happened.

Lisa died just after finding out, after months of hard work, that *The C-Word* had got a BBC One commission. There had been just enough time to do some of the writing alongside Nicole Taylor. There had been just enough time to ask Sheridan Smith to play her. Can you imagine what kind of conversation that would have been? There was, however, sadly no time to talk about how they'd round off the film, which scene would be the one that would draw it to a conclusion.

Lisa's husband Pete got in touch with me, along with the director, to talk through how we – Fran, Lisa and I – had planned to go to Brighton and toast to Ellie, another girl, same disease, who wrote about it bloody brilliantly in a blog that connected us all. Ellie had died two weeks before her wedding. It had come as a shock to us all, but particularly to me. This was the first pal death I had known and I didn't really know how to deal with it. Fran and I attended her funeral in Brixton and although it was lovely, warm, and even funny in parts, I couldn't help but feel so desperately sad. The only two people who knew exactly how it felt were Lisa and Fran. We decided we'd go to Brighton to celebrate Ellie. I'd even emailed Pete to check whether Lisa would be up for something like this, as by that point she'd already lost a lot of mobility and was using a wheelchair. He told me it would be just what she needed.

'I will throw your wheelchair in the back of my van,' I emailed. But in the end it was Fran's cancer that scuppered the plan. Yet another round of chemotherapy had failed and she needed to spend any time she did have thinking about her next move and being with her new husband, Andy. She was sorry to let us down, but I assured her we'd make it happen.

And in a way, we did. It was decided that this event, although Fran, Lisa and I never managed it, would mark the bit of the film where Lisa was coming to terms with her terminal illness, and that it would be one of the final scenes of the film. Fast-forward fifteen months, to Brighton, to my own actor's trailer, with my name on. The producers of the film asked me whether I would play myself in the film and, bearing in mind I was A) not an actress and B) shit scared, I said 'ABSOLUTELY BLOODY YES'. I even had to go along to a read-through like some kind of proper actor and go through the lines, not so much to check my skills (I think, I hope) but more to ensure that what had been scripted would have been true to life had we *actually* made it to Brighton.

'And ACTION.'

'Lisa!' I shouted towards Sheridan, who was standing at the end of Brighton Pier on a scorching-hot day in July.

The call sheet mentioned 22°C; it felt more like 50. Thank goodness for the sea breeze, which just about kept the many layers of make-up from avalanching off my face.

'It's so good to see you,' an actress called Amy, playing Fran, said as we all embraced, as per the script.

'To Anya – to life,' (Ellie's name had been changed) we toasted, with real whisky, for the third time (whether the director was just trying to get me sozzled or lighten up, I'm not sure) as I was sitting on the bum-numbing pebbles, with a wheelchair beside us and Lisa's walking stick propped against it.

We went on to improvise various chats about cancer and the ridiculous things people have said to us in the past that infuriated us or made us laugh. I was so into the pretence/drunk that I almost forgot I wasn't sitting with people who actually had cancer, who were in fact very much not dying.

That day feels as surreal now as it did then, and although I was terrified, and Sheridan did her absolute best to calm my nerves as I was trying to 'act', I was so glad and honoured to have done it, that I got a chance not to just toast to Ellie, but all three of them.

My way of coping with cancer, and in fact how fiercely I live my life, has without doubt been shaped by the many women who've walked into my life, done something to my insides, and had to leave this mortal coil way WAY before their time. I try all I can to live a life they were robbed of, to savour what they no longer get to experience (those bitches all left me before a global pandemic though didn't they – did they know something I did not?). I have taken parts of their wisdom and power along for my own ride, and without Fran, Lisa, Ellie, Giselle, Laura, Mairead, Sarah, Polly, Ciaran, Fi, Saima and Suzanne I would not be the woman I am today.

Rest in your eternal powers, ladies.

Going to the Maldives

> If the weight of mortality does not grow lighter, does
> it at least get more familiar?
>
> *Paul Kalanithi*, When Breath Becomes Air

Not only had Faye, my hospice consultant, offered antidepressants and suggested I start exercising, but to round things off she offered counselling, and there began my first steps into accepting that I might, at some point in the not-too-distant future, die. I had never aired feelings and thoughts and outrage like it until I sat in a room with a stranger and howled. She had heard it all before. Nothing shook her – however much I threw at her, she never shed a tear! No one had so casually seen through my hollow stoicism before. Anyone I'd ever shared fears with before had got upset, so this was so new and *so* refreshing to me. I was allowed to be scared, I was allowed to be really, really angry and I was allowed to take off my positivity mask that I tried to wear too much and too often, even when I really didn't need to. I allowed my outsides to match my insides. I learnt that the fears I was harbouring were way more powerful if not given a voice.

My counsellor taught me that there is value in loneliness, sadness, in unshiny feelings, and made me realise how exhausting the constant 'overcoming' had become. I realised the impact that other people's reactions to my illness were having on me. How I fed off every person who told me I 'didn't look unwell' (and I genuinely didn't, apart from during active IV chemotherapy) without realising that this invalidated my very real illness because it didn't present itself the way everyone expected it to. She made reassuring and well-timed noises and I left each session feeling a thousand times lighter, able to skip out of there ready to crack on with life. I needed to dump everything that I didn't have time or energy or mind space to deal with there in that little cosy room in Hampstead. In that time I had an epiphany: talking about death wouldn't bring it on any faster. I will repeat it again so it sinks into your brain too: TALKING ABOUT DEATH DOESN'T BRING IT ON FASTER. The moment that penny dropped I lost 100 lbs of tummy-churning anxiety.

Even before cancer, death, in more general terms, was not unfamiliar to me. I first realised that life can end abruptly when I was fifteen, when Nanna, my mum's mum, died suddenly. She was everything you'd hope a nanna to be: full of love, pride and cuddles. She gave the best cuddles because she just always seemed to be warm. She and my grandad used to pick the three of us up from school, squished into their old Rover, and the best thing about that was the sweetie tin. You weren't really ever sure what you might choose and on too many occasions I picked a humbug, which I detest to this day. Whoever thought mint and caramel make a good combo needs their head testing. Nanna and Grandad would treat us a lot and give us weekly pocket money because Mum couldn't afford to on top of paying to keep a roof over our heads. I'd usually spend that on sweets at Woolworths pick 'n' mix or on those mini drinks cans, you know the ones with Mr Blobby on.

When we first moved to England we lived with our grandparents for about six months before we could afford to move into our house in the nearby town and closer to school. The way Nanna died was the cruellest. She'd only just had a pacemaker fitted to sort out a problem that caused her to blank out and fall. Within twenty-four hours of returning home after the operation, my mum found her dead in her bed. We'd been so hopeful that she was now fixed and would have her life back in her again. I'd spent the evening before she died with her, showing off a new top I'd bought at New Look, which she loved. I loved it when she was happy and had colour in her cheeks. The moment I found out she was dead was, I guess, quite a turning point. I'd never felt such grief and sadness ever before; not even moving countries and having to start my life all over again came close.

The day it happened I was home for lunch during a work-experience week at an abrasives company (yeah, all the other slightly more fun work-experience posts were gone. While everyone else got to play with pets at the vet's surgery or watch films all day at the cinema, I got to learn the difference between lap mops and flat wheels at a firm that made sandpaper). The one benefit of working there was that it was close to home, so I could pop back for lunch. That day I thought it was strange that no one was home, but I knew Mum might be checking Nanna was settling in OK back in her house after being discharged from the hospital. I gave her a call to check in.

'I wish you hadn't called,' Mum said.

'Why?' I asked, puzzled.

'Nanna died last night.'

And that was it. My legs gave way and I crumpled into a heap on the sofa. I buried my face so hard that all I saw was black. I couldn't understand how she'd been so full of life just hours before and now gone. Completely gone. I'd literally never get to see her smile, hear her voice, feel her warmth EVER again. As well as not computing the fact I'd never see her again, I also couldn't fathom how this would ever be OK. How would I ever not be heartbroken? How could I ever think of her without crying? I guess these are questions that go around the head of anyone who has experienced the death of someone close to them. For fifteen-year-old Kris it was a lesson she wasn't ready for. How can anyone ever be ready? No amount of guinea pig or hamster deaths prepared me, that's for sure.

Everything about the days and weeks that followed Nanna's death was horrific too. My poor grandad, who had suffered a stroke four years before, had developed dementia, so we constantly had to tell him that Nanna had died. We broke his world into pieces over and over again. I got to see her body in the hospital but instantly regretted it. I had not had the chance to say goodbye to her, but seeing her lying cold and lifeless did not help in the slightest. Her funeral was horrendous and sad and the weeks helping to clear out her house, as Grandad couldn't live there on his own, were torturous too. There's a CD I bought around that same time that I would listen to over and over again. It was called *The Album* and featured tunes from Supergrass to Richard Ashcroft. Every time I hear 'Closing Time' by Semisonic, I am transported to a time when I was trying to figure out how life could be so unfair. The lyrics about each new beginning coming from some other beginning's end spoke to me.

It didn't help that those thoughts were colliding with puberty and the general feelings of melancholia that come with turning sixteen. Since I was a small girl, my biggest fear was Mum dying, and every time I saw her upset I couldn't help but imagine the pain she was in, losing her mum. In fact, it conjured memories of a night in Germany when I actually thought Mum had died. In reality she had passed out at the sight of her own blood (she's useless with blood) after cutting herself on a broken glass following a big argument with Dad and her parents. She was perched on the toilet and suddenly I saw her eyes roll to the back of her head, and I thought that was it, I'd lost her. For ever. Not understanding what fainting was, I screamed and howled inconsolably as my dad splashed cold water on Mum's face to revive her and my grandparents tried to calm me down. The imprint of that moment has lasted till now.

What I learned about Nanna's death didn't really help me when I got to experience it again five years later. It was just a pretty normal day in March 2006. The house phone rang. I answered. It was more than likely going to be someone for Mum, perhaps an English family member or a friend from Germany. I always had to ensure my German brain was vaguely switched on so if there was someone speaking German on the other end of the line I could at least say, 'Yeah, I'll just get her.' It was my German aunty. She sounded really off and not her usual jovial self and immediately asked to speak to Mum. To this day I can't work out why she thought Dad's ex-wife should find out he had died before one of his twenty-year-old daughters, but let's just say the Hallenga family weren't ones for dealing with anything in the way normal people would. My aunty told Mum that my dad had been found dead in his house by the lady who lived in the flat below him. After we moved to England, he turned the house I grew up in into two flats, as he didn't need as much space. As horrific as it was for a frail old lady to find a dead man clutching his chest at the bottom of the stairs beside the washing basket of clothes he was presumably taking to hang outside, I do wonder how long he'd have been there if she hadn't discovered him. He'd suffered a massive heart attack and it's unlikely, even with some intervention, that he would have survived it.

Sadly, it wasn't completely unexpected. My dad drank too much, smoked too much, but would also pound his heart with exercise at the gym and on his bike cycling to and from the school where he worked. As a young girl I remember visiting him in hospital rehab (something the Germans do impeccably well is ensuring people get proper rehabilitation after any operation; they call it *die Kur* – literally 'the cure') after he'd had an operation to unclog an artery in his leg, there thanks to years and years of smoking. He was warned at that point that if he didn't stop smoking, he would probably not live to see his grandchildren. Did he stop? Did he fuck. He'd spend hours on end in his office at home chain-smoking and working away on his home videos. I didn't know my dad without a camera attached to his hand. Every move we made as kids, he'd document it. However grateful I am for now having that footage doesn't really make up for the desperation you can see in our eyes, longing for our dad to put the camera down and actually play with us. In one such scene you can hear us calling his name repeatedly and, because he didn't like talking while filming, he stayed silent.

One of the many questions I'd ask him if he wasn't, ya know, dead, would be why he thought it was necessary to hide behind a camera so much. He destroyed any opportunity to connect and bond with us, which ultimately hindered any love I ever felt for him. My hatred for smoking and smokers (if you know me, you know how un-fun I can be at parties explaining to smokers why it's a shit habit. Yup, I'm that person) stems purely from the anger and frustration I experienced via Mum and then later for myself. Maren and I would stick plasters over the keyhole to his office so that the stench didn't enter the rest of the house.

The Christmas before he died, Maren and I decided to send him an ultimate plea asking him to stop smoking. By this point we were only seeing him about two or three times a year, if we visited during our or his school or uni breaks. We wrote him a letter asking him to stop so that he was still around to walk us down an aisle – more emotional blackmail than a real threat, since neither of us actually thought we'd get married, but, ya know, we had to hit him where it might hurt. We told him he ran a big risk of never seeing his grandchildren. That should do it, we thought.

His reply came with a promise to stop. Finally he admitted that it was time to quit smoking and that he needed help in doing so. Four months later he was dead. It was too little, too late – in fact, he hadn't even kept his promise, because on entering his flat for the first time after he died, we found numerous packets of fags and a well-stocked booze cupboard. He was never not in self-destruction mode: at least, that's how I saw it as a child and how I saw it when he died, only later realising that he was clearly struggling with every addiction going – with alcohol, with sex, with smoking. My first memory of him is no different from the final one of him, and what's most sad is that when he died I lost the opportunity to ever change how I feel about him.

I so wish I could speak to him now and try to understand why he chose to do the many stupid things he did. I recognise some of his characteristics in myself. He was liked (by people other than his wife), confident and had loads of friends – so many friends they didn't all fit in the church at his funeral. But he, like me, often didn't really think things through fully, often didn't communicate his decision-making or make it clear how he really felt, perhaps sometimes opting for a head-in-sand approach instead of dealing with problems. The days leading up to his funeral were full of endless revelations and disappointments. We found out he owed money to relatives, had a porn habit, loose threads and no sign of a will. He left us with a pile of shit to deal with. There was no evidence he had *ever* considered his own death, and *boy*, have I learned from that mistake.

So many people that I'd never met before, from students to colleagues and choir buddies, were singing his praises, and all I could think was, *Are we at the right funeral?* I wasn't experiencing any of this alone, of course: Mum, Maike, Maren and I were all making these discoveries together. We could laugh till we cried about it all. Our collective anguish, confusion and bewilderment helped us get through those days before the funeral. The only time we didn't discuss and mull over his dumb life decisions was on the way to the church. I remember Imogen Heap's 'Hide and Seek' was playing from one of our many mixtapes. All you O.C. fans will remember that this very tune was played as people arrived at Caleb's funeral, so it had an even greater impact on an emo like me. Later, as the three of us spoke the words of the classic, unoriginal funeral poem 'Do Not Stand at My Grave and Weep' by Mary Elizabeth Frye, I wanted so badly to believe he was that version of a great man everyone else seemed to be remembering. The only thing that made it any better was the cake – in Germany most funerals involve *Freud-und-Leid-Kuchen* ('joy and sorrow cake'), also known as *Beerdigungskuchen* ('funeral cake') – a buttery sponge cake topped with sugar and flaked almonds and more sugar and more butter. It's one thing I give Germans props for: trying to make an otherwise hideous day a bit better with cake made out of tons of butter and sugar, the best way to drown any sorrows.

To this day I hold on to regrets about my relationship with my dad. I don't feel the standard grief surrounding my dad's death; I think I grieve for a relationship I didn't get to have. I'm sad that I never got to understand him better and ask him where and why it all went so wrong with my mum. I've heard her side of the story many times; in fact, her side was all I knew and understood as we moved to England. There's no skirting around the fact that he was a philanderer, but what was it about being with Mum and having us that just wasn't enough? I've obviously learned to ease off on the anguish of never knowing and focus instead on ensuring my death is absolutely nothing like his: nothing left unsaid, no pile of crap to sort, no debt.

Experiencing the deaths of my nanna, my dad, friends and cat taught me about loss but not my own mortality – it would be cancer that did that. Grief has allowed me to reach some emotional depths that I didn't know existed, and allowed my perspective on life to shift, but it's not until I faced my own mortality that the real 'ah-ha' moments happened. Grieving someone and facing my own mortality are very different and in a way I feel privileged to get to experience both. Grief is proof I loved, that something or someone meant something to me, moved me, and made my life richer. It's hard – *fuck*, it's hard – but it reminds me how lucky I am to feel. Death is different.

Facing my mortality has been harder to accept than having the disease itself. Who in their early twenties, and now thirties, can ever *really* be OK with dying? Sometimes the enormity of my situation sucks the breath out of me. Sometimes I am so riddled with fear that nothing makes sense any more. I fear a painful death. I fear the suffering. I also fear the nothingness that death brings. The complete and utter void. The unknown. It's why I respect and envy those who have faith in an afterlife; surely that must bring some comfort. I don't have that. Is it weird that the only way I have found to cope with the fear of death is thinking about and exploring it?

I might not have control of when it happens, but I've still considered on many occasions what might be the best way to die. Is it better to leave without warning, no goodbye, no long-drawn-out ending, like my nanna and dad? Or to have a diagnosis that will almost certainly end in death, whether that's within weeks or years? I still haven't really fully decided; my thinking on this remains fluid. What I do appreciate is that I've even had time to consider this. I have been given an opportunity to prepare for my death and get my head around the idea of a 'good death'. Yeah, I too thought that was a bit of an oxymoron at first, but let me tell you how I think it's possible. A good death starts with understanding that it's possible to have a full and meaningful good life. Being prepared for life to end already gives you a head start in understanding it's possible to end it all well – as my good friend, and well-known speaker and writer, Sophie Sabbage once said, 'It is possible to RIP *before* you die.' In allowing myself to consider what a good death might look like and acknowledging it and welcoming it, rather than letting it fester somewhere deep in my head, I've found a calm place. Also, there are benefits of actively knowing you are going to die: you get to see the fruit of your life. I've managed to reflect on stuff with greater respect and without it I'm not sure I would have come to the conclusion that I'm actually a pretty good egg.

I was once given a session with a conscious dying expert named Richard over Skype. Not your average call, but my fascination for all things death was peaking. I don't really know why I thought it was necessary to confront death that particular day or week or month, but I wanted to use the opportunity to air my thoughts on my own death and potentially learn something new. Richard had a varied job background ranging from support-worker roles, physiotherapy and also the ambulance service before moving on to dying expert. It was the moments he spent in the back of an ambulance that made him turn to helping people deal with dying. Whenever someone was panicking about potential imminent death, he observed that the paramedics would try to calm them with, 'Let's not talk like that,' or, 'We won't let you die,' which would shut the patient up but instead leave them all alone with their thoughts of dying. Had they been allowed to express and acknowledge an end to their life, they might have aired wishes and thoughts they wanted to pass on. It goes without saying that paramedics are not death doulas – they are there to get someone to hospital and ensure they don't die on the way – but Richard felt uneasy about it all. To him, ignorance wasn't always bliss. Some of them were indeed dying, and we will all face that very same fate, yet we fail to see that acknowledging what is happening makes it easier for ourselves and others. He also taught me that we go through life dealing with different losses all the time – the loss of a job, relationship, health, identity. The way we deal with those things ultimately shapes how we deal with our death.

My favourite The Chicks songs are playing, there is soft lighting from candles (posh ones), Lady M is purring gently at the end of the bed, a friend is massaging my feet (poor sod), pals are playing Dobble (or Shit or Sausage – google it), there is belly laughter, my old home-town friend Stacey is ensuring I get no sympathy, Niall is being inappropriate, I am pain-free but not so off my non-existent tits that I'm barely conscious and/or dribbling, there are snacks (gelato, crisps), there is wine (Malbec), there are frames with photo memories, there is trash talk, there is thoughtful silence. There is peace. There is closure. I'm not describing my perfect Sunday afternoon, although gladly I'd do all this weekly – I'm imagining, and picturing and manifesting, if you will, my perfect death scenario. Much like a birth plan, it's possible to have a death plan, and although many circumstances may scupper this all, it still feels good to imagine what a relatively pain-free, peaceful end could look like because I know that through engaging in death, it doesn't have to be – NEWSFLASH – as horrific, tragic and dramatic as it is in films. I've read so many books on the subject from *Do Death* by Amanda Blainey and *We All Know How This Ends* by Anna Lyons and Louise Winter to *When Breath Becomes Air* by Paul Kalanithi and *With the End in Mind* by Kathryn Mannix. I read *Being Mortal* by Atul Gawande on the beach in Portugal and so many pennies dropped; the more facts I knew, the less I was guessing and fearing.

Thanks to the hospice, I've made an advanced care plan that sets out my plans A and B for where I'd like to die. I can be as prescriptive and specific as I like, even down to telling others what sort of music I might like playing, or what interventions, if any, I'd like them to carry out to make me comfortable. We get one crack at this dying malarkey and I can tell you that as much as I have needed to gain control of my life, I need to ensure I don't relinquish an iota of it until my last breath! I want to decide when enough is enough, and I hope I have the strength and mental stability to do that. I don't want to keep going for the sake of it. I don't want to hang on because society has taught us all that anyone with cancer has to 'fight' until the bitter end. In fact, guys, I'm calling bullshit on that. Saying you've had enough is not failure. LET ME REPEAT: saying you've had enough is not failure. It's just as brave and OK to say, '*Enough*,' and to 'fight' no more. Death is not a failure. It's not a test: we don't succeed or fail at it.

It's OK for the doctor – your doctor – to be honest and say that more drugs, especially the ones with all the side effects, are probably making no impact now and instead focus should be made on comfort and quality end-of-life time. I say this with such ease and yes, things might be different, and I may crumble and deny and defy, but this moment, when I am well, is when I can hope for the best-case scenario. I've known friends who knew when enough was enough, who bravely decided when they stopped all treatment to savour whatever quality time they had away from hospital. I also know of friends who endured drugs until their very last breath, more for their families' sake than their own. I don't know how I will feel about treatments when I'm nearing the end, but there is power in letting go. There is control in saying 'no more'. I've even taken it one step further by putting in place a lasting power of attorney for my health as well as my wealth, so if or when I can no longer make decisions with a clear mind, my twin sister, legally, can. We're not talking about who my many properties and assets are left to because, well, I don't have any; it's purely to make the ending and aftermath that bit less stressful. I have my dad and all his baggage to thank for that.

To some extent I have control, but there is something I can't command once I'm gone. I'm not talking about the funeral – that I've thought about and planned too (partly because I cannot face the idea of my family calling the random funeral parlour person on the high street with dusty curtains and fake flowers in the window); for example, I want a cheap and eco-friendly coffin to be cremated in, and potted plants for people to take home, not cut ones. I want 'Cloud Number Nine' by Bryan Adams playing at some point to fulfil the wishes of ten-year-old Kris. There's more, but you don't need to know it all; it's noted somewhere for those who need to see it. What I can't control is how I am remembered, how people will talk about my death, and me. Will it be laced with tragedy? Will people focus more on how I died, rather than how I lived? I don't want the number of years I was alive to overshadow what I crammed into them. I hope no one will say I have 'lost my battle'. To say I have lost anything would undo all my hard work building and sustaining a life that I loved and valued and squeezed all the goodness out of. I would like to think that people have witnessed that I live with greater authenticity, candour and gratitude, that I have cultivated a true lust for life.

I want to be remembered as someone who valued simplicity. I don't need people to say how much I achieved; I need them to point out how happy I was to simply be and how I made them feel (I mean, hopefully good). Fuck, I think that will be my greatest legacy. Why does that matter? Well, I think there's unfathomable pressure on cancer patients to make the most out of every single bloody day. To some extent I agree, but it's not that sustainable, is it? It feeds a constant 'I should be grateful and making the most out of life' conundrum. When my house needs cleaning, I should be grateful that I've been alive long enough for my toilet to even get dirty and for the floor to need vacuuming. But that doesn't mean it's going to get clean by itself.

Someone once asked me in an interview if I thought women could 'have it all'. By all I could only assume she meant a family and, *shock*, a career. But I challenged her on this. The 'all' is surely subjective. My 'all' is simple: to just be. Your all could be sheep shearing in the Outer

Hebrides with a pet pig. Your 'all' is exactly that: *yours*, no matter what pressures society, interviewers or Instagram put on you. Just remember to simply put 'being' at the centre of your 'all'. That's why I don't have a bucket list. I want connections, not things. Bucket lists are for people who haven't found what makes them happy right now. Being more mindful and OK with simplicity ensures I don't long for more. Not having a bucket list gets rid of the pressure to see, do, achieve, experience stuff that I might never get to do. Death makes you challenge all of the things you *want*, and reminds you of the things you already *have*. Do I want to lie on my deathbed wishing I'd made it to the Grand Canyon? Nope. Do I want to feel like I'm content with everything I did do because I experienced it fully, richly and wholly? *Yup*. Take the focus off quantity and hone in on quality. It's the only way I've found peace with the fact my life may end sooner than most. I want to be *that* smug bitch on my deathbed.

The longer I have cancer the more I realise that the small things in life are actually the big things. Most of life is made up of everyday connections, big bright moons, blossom, laughing, fresh coffee and handwritten letters – the everyday constants. Big things are fun, but I doubt they will be what I will want to remember about my wonderful life. I want to honour my life and the people in my life. If I do die tomorrow, I can be happy and not regret how I lived today. (Is this the place to admit that I'm not sure I've eaten enough gelato, had enough sex or tried hallucinogenics yet?)

So, I don't expect you to get yourself a conscious dying expert (in fact, you can learn all you need to know about death from a great Disney film called *Coco*) and I'm not saying you should rush to write a will or fill out a lasting power of attorney right now (but soon?); what I need you to do is simply have a chat with someone you love about dying, about their fears, their wishes, their remaining hopes and possible regrets. Ask yourself and each other how you want to die, if you want a funeral, what special wishes you/they have. Let that shit out and prepare for something you might not expect: a will to live on and then probs a full dishwasher that needs emptying.

Here are some things I bet you didn't know to end this chapter:

- You can be buried in your own garden (there are, of course, some rules!).
- You don't have to have a funeral.
- Funerals don't have to cost the earth, no matter how much the adverts on daytime telly try to convince you otherwise.
- You don't need to be removed from your home (if you've died there) until your loved ones are ready.

- It doesn't have to be dramatic and awful like in the movies.
- There are no rules for when you live or die or say goodbye.
- I can have my dead cat's ashes cremated *with* me when I die.
- You *can* RIP before you die.

Imposter Syndrome with a Floppy Hat

It's a sunny day in July 2015 and I'm standing in the Arkwright Building at Nottingham Trent University. A citation has just been read about me and all my work with CoppaFeel!, and I'm now standing and walking towards a podium to accept an honorary doctorate in public administration and to share some words of wisdom with graduating students. I'm wearing the most colourful outfit and a floppy hat with a tassel. I'm sweating so much. I open my mouth . . .

Chancellor/Vice-Chancellor, ladies and gentlemen, people with boobs . . .

Thank you so much for this recognition. This is an incredible honour and I cannot even begin to explain how happy it makes me or even expect anyone to understand. To understand, you too would have had to be diagnosed with incurable cancer, endured hellish treatments, started a charity, worked your ass off and still doubted yourself immeasurably. But since I don't recommend you get cancer, I can't make you realise how this feels. It's moments like this that make me want to live more than anything and remind me why being alive is pretty freaking cool.

I never expected to find myself giving advice to people graduating from an establishment of higher education, because I never graduated from one of these myself. It wasn't for me, because there was nothing I felt passionate about, nothing that moved me enough, until of course I was diagnosed with breast cancer and discovered that young people were not getting the cancer education they needed. I couldn't imagine living in the world where people weren't given the best chance to survive this insidious disease, so in a sense I didn't have a choice but to do something about it, and therein I found my passion, my reason, and an unshakable and heady conviction that I would, maybe, change the world.

I wanted to share some nuggets of wisdom with you. Stuff I've learned that may serve as advice:

1. *When I started CoppaFeel! I had no idea what I was doing; in fact, I still don't. But I learned by doing and blagging. And you know what?*

Anything that's easy isn't worth it! Where would be the fun in doing something guaranteed to work?

2. *There will be days when you think the world is conspiring against you. At that point don't underestimate the power of a good cup of tea. And* Neighbours *– and no I don't mean the people who live next door to you (although they might be able to help too), I mean the TV show. And if that's no use, CRY. It's OK to cry (that goes for you boys too!). Be there for others, listen and be ready to stick the kettle on.*

3. *YOU and only you are responsible for your own happiness. Don't blame others: happiness and good fortune won't be handed to you on a plate.*

4. *Mary Poppins was right: fun is non-negotiable.*

5. *There's a world out there starving for good leadership that craves your wisdom, your creativity and your humanity. Go be good people, because the world needs you. And if you don't know how, just pretend to be someone who does.*

6. *Something that you have that nobody has is YOU. Live, dance, travel, explore, ask questions, LOVE like only you can.*

7. *Spend less time on your phone, look up, look around you, press PLAY on life.*

I am here on this very stage for a reason, and if cancer is the reason then so be it. YOU are here for a reason: you have worked hard and we're here to celebrate your efforts.

Whether you pursued tertiary education to follow your dream or please your parents, I hope you know how privileged you are to have been given the opportunity to learn. You are ready and able to do beautiful things in this world! Recognise your passion, feel it, and go make the world a more interesting and better place.

I may have lost a boob and the chance of a long life, but what I have gained is pretty awesome – I mean, HELLO, an honorary doctorate!!!! – but ya know what? It shouldn't take a cancer diagnosis to do epic things and make a good mark on the world. Go and own your meaning with or without cancer. Make. Shit. Happen.

And lastly, because it's my job to, I must also

remind you to go check your boobs tonight. And I mean your own.

Have a wonderful day. See you on the dance floor . . .

I shut my mouth. I sit down. I hear applause. I look up at my beaming family in an ocean of bobbing mortarboards and proud parent grins.

Time to Sharpen My Saw

It is amazing what you can accomplish if you do not
care who gets the credit.

Harry S. Truman

I stretched, yawned and sunk back into my soft duvet.
Wilhelm, woken by my leg movement, greeted me with a
gentle paw prod. We were in our new little house in
Cornwall, a mere hop, skip and a jump from the ocean.
The ocean to and into which I could escape when life felt
a bit much. When I dunk myself in the water I am
immediately brought back inside my body and it's like
I'm in a time outside of time, where all of the world's
problems don't exist. That weightlessness is both sooth-
ing for my achy body and achy soul. The seagulls
squawked, signalling either bin-collection day or a cheery
'*Welcome to Cornwall, Kris*'. I decided it was the latter.

I had decided a few months earlier that my time in
London was up. The tenancy on the flat I moved into in

Hackney after Catface and I broke up was nearing the end, and my flatmate Rach was heading to pastures new too. Six years in London is just about the right amount of time before you start to hate it or potentially never leave. I didn't see myself in London forever – I mean, actually I hadn't really seen at all into the future, but I visited Maren in Cornwall whenever I could and always felt a sense of calm there that I never could in London. She was living in a village near Newquay. I wasn't prepared to relinquish *all* the conveniences I had in London, such as being walking distance from a shop, so I settled on living in a friend's rented little house in Newquay itself, with a big bedroom window from where I could, if the wind was blowing in the right direction and I focused very intensely, hear the sea roaring.

Maren had already taken a back seat from the charity a year before and was pursuing design work. Now it was my turn and my time to perhaps, I dunno, breathe a bit – physically and mentally – away from London. I'd made the decision to step down as CEO of CoppaFeel! and here are some reasons why:

1. My plan was never to run the charity forever. The best thing I learned was to have an exit plan, because that means you have got the organisation to a place where it can exist without you. I'd always dreamed of the day when I didn't have to

worry about the charity. A bit like (well, nothing like it, but hear me out) parents dreaming of the day when they can go to sleep without checking on their baby through the night. I wanted to see my baby grow up, flourish and for me to move on. It helped knowing and seeing how much I'd already achieved. We were conducting annual market research that told us that if people had heard of CoppaFeel! they were more likely to check their boobs regularly. And not as meaningful, but still a big deal for me: we were now in our own offices with our own doorbell and our own kettle (but in my heart our charity will remain small and scrappy forever, I think).

2. I wanted control – had you guessed by now that I like control? I think it stemmed from never really ever trusting myself and finding it very hard to trust others. But that was changing. However, I wanted to be the one who decided when I stopped working for CoppaFeel!, *not* cancer. I dreaded the conversation I might one day have to have with our team about my inability to carry on leading because cancer was forcing me to stop; that I was too weak, too ill to be a CEO any more. God, the thought of that makes me shiver. I had started the charity professionally, keeping cancer and my

work life separate; I wanted that to continue until the day I died.

3. It had been seven years of me running the show. I was no longer doing the fun stuff: the creative big ideas, the face-to-face chats in a field. Managing people and dramas became an almost daily activity. I'm not a manager: I'm an ideas girl, a doer; I'm not a natural leader of a pack (I obviously had to be, but that doesn't mean I was the best at it). The charity needed a strong CEO to take it to the next level. In every organisation there's a vast treasure trove of untapped high-quality leadership lying dormant, and it's the job of any leader to release that hidden leadership, not to keep it bottled up, unused. Our marketing and brand director Nat rose to the challenge and has been bossing the role since. I'd done the groundwork; it was time for me to sit back. What a great feeling that was. What a privilege. All my hard work had led to that sense of relief. I could let go of that control. I had learned that too much control leaves no wriggle room, no space for trust. I was trusting myself and in turn trusted others too.

4. Founders shouldn't run charities forever, because they run the risk of sucking the life out of them.

With a trustee board that still had founding members, I could trust our original ethos and culture wouldn't be going anywhere any time soon. But for our strategy I never wanted to reach a feeling of comfort because, as my pal Dave Cornthwaite once said, 'Comfort kills ambition.' I didn't want that. To me the focus was: make the most effective contribution you can, then retire graciously.

5. Your value on Planet Earth is not calculated by your productivity. For so long I had placed cancer and productivity at war with one another, feeling that the more time I gave to cancer, the less I could achieve. There was always another email to write. Always another smile to smile. It was time for me to really learn how to 'be' and unlearn the constant need to 'do'. I would still be employed by the charity, but part time, doing ambassadorial jobs, working with our amazing patrons and, of course, still organising Festifeel, because that was something I still held on to dearly. It was, and still is, the one thing that sparks my creativity and joy and brings together the real essence of our charity.

6. My identity was rooted in cancer. It was scary to let go of something that had felt safe. But it was

time to discover whether cancer had made me brave enough to unlock even more of myself. Perhaps there wasn't more, and that would be fine, but I was keen to know for sure. For seven years my heart and soul had been consumed by little else but CoppaFeel!, and now I needed to make space for other stuff too.

Although I had moved all my belongings and my life to Cornwall, my medical team were still in London, and before I knew it I was back in that Charing Cross Hospital waiting room with my friend Simon. It wasn't unusual to have to wait for over an hour to see an oncologist, but even when things were more swift and on time, I still hated it there, hospital time was dead time. The air always felt thicker, the atmosphere so gloomy, not helped by the abstract art on the walls that did nothing to lift my spirits, only confuse my mind – perhaps that was its purpose, to distract us poor patients from possible bad news once entering a magnolia-coloured room. The only time this place was a nice place to be was when my pal Sarah joined me with treats and flowers that she handed out to very confused and actually not that grateful patients in the waiting room. Eventually I got called in to see Dr Hope.

'I need to have a think. I have a lot of plans this summer, including a trip to Italy and then a hike in Iceland for

CoppaFeel! Oh, and also Maren and I are thinking of buying a vintage truck and turning it into a coffee-and-cake mobile café.'

Probably not the reaction you'd expect from someone who had been told their cancer was on the move yet again and therefore a more aggressive, according to my oncologist, treatment plan was needed. His response: 'You need to be alive to do those things.'

Something told me in that moment my time with this oncologist had run its course. I had swapped oncologists before; I knew I could do it again. His words, delivered without even looking me in the eyes, hit me harder than any had in a while. 'You need to be alive to do those things.' I'd been plodding along OK. It had been two years since we last discovered some activity – another brain tumour, which we had treated the same way as the one in 2012, with very targeted stereotactic radio-therapy. The tumour was once again tiny, not causing me any symptoms, and was only picked up by a routine scan. The rest of the cancer in my body was behaving, or as he had come to call it, 'dead pigeon-like', so we had made the decision to stay on track with the treatment I was already on.

I'd *always* appreciated Dr Hope's attitude to treatment – to not jump straight into the sledgehammer approach. To move gently, gently. Until now, that is. Now the tumours in my liver had suddenly become less dead pigeon-like and more sort of flapping around, making themselves known. Without the scans you wouldn't be able to tell, though – I was still looking and feeling well. So now he wanted me to enter a trial that he had designed, which involved IV chemotherapy alongside a hormone drug. The chemo was a pretty tough one called eribulin, and my two references in that moment of this treatment were: 1) friends trying it as a last-ditch resort before sadly dying and 2) hearing a sales pitch from a drug rep about it at a recent talk I gave to clinicians. Of course I needed time to think; it had been seven years, and by now I truly knew not to rush into any decisions about treatment. I knew that, contrary to popular belief, I did have time to process and research my next steps, and I had every right to say to him, 'I'll think about it.'

His reaction and pushiness really disappointed me and now here I was, having to make decisions about my next treatment steps once again. I kept having to ask Simon whether he too was taken aback by Dr Hope's approach. Was he having a bad day? Why would he dangle death in front of my face like that? Was he so desperate for an applicant to his trial that he was using such harsh tactics? He had been my doctor for five years and I had placed all my trust in him and his approach, and now I felt alone again.

I cried a lot. I cried waiting for the train at the station. I cried hopeless tears of exhaustion. When I mustered the energy to go to the office, I cried there too. I knew if I could just grab onto something positive, some tiny little noodle of hope that things would be OK, then I'd be OK and could think of something other than how my life felt balanced on a thin line again, and how I had to find a solution again. I had to dig deep. You might think that by now I'd be used to tapping into some very deep resolve to get through the day, but in all honesty, the decision about which treatment or tactic to try next consumed me. I was teetering on the edge of making possibly the worst decision ever – the fact that I'd previously made the right decisions about my care didn't reassure me one iota. I was swivelling wildly between trusting my gut instinct that this wasn't right for me – it had stood me in good stead before – and putting my faith in Dr Hope's medical integrity.

Experience had taught me that I didn't have to go with the first possible solution to the current problem. Now you may think this is a case of a desperate person who would stop at nothing to find someone who would say what they wanted to hear, but I have a long-term commitment to finding a space between hopelessness and delusion. I read the pamphlet about the trial Dr Hope wanted me to participate in, going over and over the details and the purpose, and, genuinely, nothing sat right with me. It didn't seem right to jump into an aggressive chemotherapy with some hefty side effects when we'd managed to avoid it since 2009. I was feeling well, and apart from the scan, nothing indicated I was any worse than before the results chat. I know that doesn't necessarily mean that bad things aren't brewing beneath the surface. According to the scan, my liver tumours were growing and my cancer markers – tested every month alongside a normal blood count – indicated that something was awry. In March I'd had my ovaries taken out – called an oophorectomy – in a bid to rid my body of producing any cancer food, a.k.a. oestrogen. My shrivelled little egg-producing prunes had packed up and left the building when I started hormone treatment from day one, but there was still a small risk they were producing something of use to cancer. It wasn't a big op, not even a night in hospital – the air they pumped me with was the most painful bit about it, resolved only by walking around my flat and farting lots. *Why*, having been through that, didn't it do the trick and halt any new growth? That's a rhetorical question, because if we knew the answer to that, we'd have a lot of lives spared.

Enter stage left my friend Maddie, who worked for a pharmaceutical company, she had done some digging to find out who might be a good second opinion in oncology in Cornwall. I scoffed at the idea at first. *As if* there'd be someone in Cornwall who could have better solutions than my *top-of-the-range* oncologist in London. *As if* any self-respecting oncologist would even practise in Cornwall if he was in any way serious about the role. I pictured some long-haired shorts-wearing surfer dude rocking up to the clinic with a surfboard under his arm with the nonchalance of a teenager.

'I've spoken to a few colleagues: HE'S YOUR MAN,' she wrote in capitals on a WhatsApp message.

Never one to doubt suggestions such as these – especially not from Maddie – I set about arranging a meeting with said hippie surfer – I mean, doctor. I hadn't actually planned to move my treatment to Cornwall; I was more than prepared to keep my cancer care in London and keep accessing it whenever I came up for various other boob-related activities or when catching up with friends. I'd come to love the train journeys between Bodmin Parkway and Paddington. The stretch between Teignmouth and Exeter that hugged the coastline never failed to make me happy. It gave me time to work, time to dream, time to catch up on telly – seriously, you can catch up on eight episodes of *Neighbours* in that time. But now things were different.

As luck would have it, I scored myself an appointment pretty quickly, after nagging my GP for the referral. It would take another *four months* before my scan images and reports would be sent down to Cornwall; you'd think someone was sending them on the back of a turtle, not the, ya know, *very speedy* internet. Red tape and bureaucracy were sadly not new to me. Regardless, Dr

Wheatley was prepared to see *me*, not my insides on a computer screen.

Maren and I walked into the Sunrise Centre at Royal Cornwall Hospital with a multitude of questions and fears and worries and hopes about what this appointment might bring forth. At this stage, I didn't know of any conventional cancer treatment alternatives, so I wasn't sure what Dr Duncan Wheatley might suggest other than maybe a different chemo, but I held on to the hope that he might just try and savour the quality of life I had worked damned hard to find and wasn't willing to let go of any time soon – and I had that trip to Italy and Iceland ahead of me, remember. He asked me the usual questions around my diagnosis and I shared them for what felt like the millionth time, and then he concerned himself with my personal life, my living set-up. Really, I just wanted him to tell me he had some magical cure – yup, seven years knowing that this does not exist doesn't stop your mind wishing for it, OK!

'So, tell me about this chemo and hormone combo trial you've been offered.'

I told him what I knew.

'It sounds odd. I think you either try chemo or you don't. It doesn't make sense to me to try it in combination with something else.'

'OK.' Hope was building.

'You don't need to do chemo just yet. We have other options and we may as well exhaust them and leave chemo on the shelf until we need it.'

There it was. That noodle of OK-ness that I needed *so* badly. He offered me everolimus (known as a targeted therapy because it wallops one cancer receptor in particular) in combination with exemestane (another hormonal therapy). I went on to tell him about how I had already started looking into some integrative drugs and tactics (more on that later). I thought I'd start this relationship off honestly: lay out on the table that I would not hide stuff from him.

'You could waltz in here chewing on a dandelion but it's not for me to tell you not to. This is your life. I give you my options, what I can offer you, and you have the right to turn them down.' I allowed myself a wry smile.

Bingo. He was indeed my man. He got me; he knew this was life. We'd established what I now tell everyone with cancer to establish: a partnership.

I can't express enough how important the doctor–patient relationship and partnership is. The thing that gets me questioning is a doctor who warns me not to think or question. I won't passively outsource my trust in my body and my own survival. If at any point since my initial diagnosis I no longer felt that I was part of the team, that I was merely an NHS number, I knew I would need to change course. It wasn't enough to have a doctor I got along with, who asked the odd question about my home life; what I needed too was the ability, the breathing space and the confidence to ask *why* and the balls to say, 'No, that's not for me.' Oh, and to not have to come into the hospital for 'catch-ups' when they could be done on the phone to save me the anguish of the waiting room.

What I also need is:

- To never worry about taking up too much time.
- To be able to ask to see the doctor again about anything I'm unsure about.
- To not be afraid to ask what they hope the outcome will be from said treatment or procedure – remember, knowledge is power.
- To remember I don't need to make decisions on the spot.
- To be aware and accept that with cancer there are no specifics and no guarantees.
- Never ever to have to apologise for googling stuff but also to be mindful of what I read and its source.
- To show my vulnerability.
- To have autonomy over my treatment plan.
- To be treated as an equal.

If any of the above is ever met with a hint of arrogance and a torpedo-sized ego (or, as my girlfriends like to call it, 'trumpet dick', if male) then I need to move on, honey. It took me a while to learn this, of course it did; it took some time to shake off how depleted and defeated my initial diagnosis made me feel, but it also stoked a fire in me that continually shouted 'never again'.

I was encouraged to read these words in Lawrence LeShan's *Cancer as a Turning Point* on this very subject recently:

> By and large, the more you are and stay in control of your own destiny, the better you will do. This approach may weaken the hospital staff's sense of omnipotence but before you allow people to play God with you, make sure they have the qualifications!

My greatest respect has gone to the doctors who simply say, 'I don't know.' Even better if it's followed by, 'But let's work together to find out,' but I won't be too greedy and I think I've made my point.

In the very same appointment I was also assigned a clinical nurse specialist, a CNS for short. She was shocked to hear that in my seven years of having cancer, she was my very first nurse specialist. Apparently everyone with secondary cancer is meant to have one. WHO KNEW? She is there to attend appointments, chase up scans, tests, prescriptions – basically help you with all the admin that comes with cancer. I didn't bother to question why the hell I'd never been assigned one before now – nothing to gain from that but frustration, and I was already more than aware of the vast differences between hospital trusts. Today I had a CNS. Today I had an oncologist who did happen to surf *and* mountain bike in his spare time, but who also had a plan. I told him my doubt about any decent doctors being in Cornwall. To which he said: 'We want quality of life too.' Which is, actually, a totally fair point. He did go to London, in fact he knew everyone I'd already contacted or had the pleasure of being treated by. Being the clinical research lead for the South West, he was always at conferences in London or the US or wherever the hell he needed to go to find out the latest treatments; he just happened to live in Cornwall.

I left with my heartbeat back in normal range and with a renewed faith in my medical team – and also my body. Not only was I about to move all my treatment and care to Cornwall, my route home had vastly changed too. No longer did I have to wrangle space on a crowded Tube; instead I had a quiet country lane and the occasional tractor to contend with.

I broke up with Dr Hope via email. I thanked him for the dedication and help he'd given me and genuinely shared my appreciation for the way he'd handled my care over the past five years.

Shortly after, Dr Wheatley a.k.a. Duncan managed to switch me onto a brand new drug called palbociclib. Something hot off the press, something he was only able to get me on compassionate terms. He was already proving to be the doctor I needed him to be. My mind was blown that I was taking a drug that was barely in a test tube the day I was told I had breast cancer seven years earlier. I always sneered when someone would try to cheer me up by saying, 'There's a treatment just around the corner – they are discovering new things all the time!' It was harder to believe knowing that secondary breast cancer drug research gets so little attention and invest- ment that it can feel like we've been given up on. But I was glad to be proved wrong, for now, and that I had been granted access to a new drug that was hailed as a bit of a breakthrough, with the added bonus of minimal side effects, so I could do as I had planned and sharpen my saw.

Alive to Do Those Things

I was alive (despite the horrendous new addition of mouth ulcers from my new drug regimen) to take that trip to Italy that summer with Maren. When something like cancer and its treatments threatens your existence, I can't begin to explain how good that first sip of Italian wine was, how tear-jerking every sunset was, how amazing it was to hear the sea and the soft linen curtains around my bed gently shuffling in the wind. I'd never been more relieved to get away, to have made it happen, to have listened to my gut.

I was alive to do that trek in Iceland with a group of fifty CoppaFeel! supporters and my older sister Maike. Walking 58 km across alien moon-like landscapes along the Landmannalaugar route with steep climbs and tough descents, past thundering waterfalls, steaming lava fields, plunging fjords and spouting geysers! And in the process raising over £160k for CoppaFeel!.

I was alive to buy that vintage truck with Maren, call her Beyoncé (because at the time there were twins inside the real Beyoncé, too. To us this made perfect sense) and start a new journey of baking and barista-ing. We'd only ever made pretty shit coffee on our friend's double-decker bus café at a mountain-bike event in Scotland *many* years ago, so this was a new skill. We baked and baked until we perfected our mini bundt cakes – like the classic German ones we used to get every birthday baked by our grandma, only in miniature, using different seasonal things to flavour and decorate them with. After all these years Maren and I were making our restaurant, Maki, come true, in a slightly different form, after all!

We'd take the van to different spots around Cornwall: sometimes festivals, sometimes a spot along a cycling track. We'd lose count of the number of people who'd come up to tell us that we were living *their* dream. How they too wished they could escape their current lives, move to the sea and open a food truck. My response was only ever, 'What's stopping you?'

Chewing on a Dandelion

I have always taken an integrative approach to my cancer treatment. I have paid people to touch me, prod me with needles, stick me in an oxygen chamber, give me intentional fevers, hug me and watch me cry. To start with it was pretty small scale, then ramped up later, when things got particularly scary with the cancer progression in 2016 – not sure why it had to get *even* more scary for me to *really* dig deep and find out how else I could support my body, but *there we are*. I went into research overdrive and it all pointed in the direction of a more holistic and integrative approach. This wasn't necessarily a new thing, as I had taken a – admittedly quite basic – holistic approach from the start that included frequent reflexology sessions and drinking wheatgrass powder mixed with juice – pretty gross, like swallowing a meadow – *every single morning* without fail during my first stint with chemotherapy. Oh and green tea; I still drink it religiously now. I can't be sure it's the reason my bloods were always good enough for chemo but it did me no harm either way.

Not long after I was diagnosed and just before I even started chemo, during a little getaway in Cornwall to see Maren I thought I'd go and speak to the people at the local Chinese herbal emporium. They concocted some immune-boosting tea herb mix for me, which resembled our compost bin and smelt like guinea-pig cage. One whiff and a tiny slurp had me gagging and that was the end of that. Something I was more committed to was my limiting of dairy and sugar consumption. I'd read too many things about how much cancer loves sugar, so tried to be really conscious of how much I ate at certain times. I remember so clearly a time I saw a massive billboard advert for a new KitKat, which I think had a caramel layer in it. I told myself that if my next scan was good I would treat myself to one. And when the scans were good I did indeed eat one and I can report it didn't live up to the hype.

It couldn't have been long after that my feelings towards sugar and cancer relaxed. This was not because I didn't believe the stuff I'd read and educated myself on, it was more that I took a conscious stance on how much I was willing to stop living. Extreme, I know, since we're talking about chocolate. But I *really like chocolate*. And no, you can't fob me off with 80 per cent dark stuff: it doesn't do it for me. I need Cadbury's Buttons. Or Twirls.

They make me happy – happier than the guilt I felt about eating sugar. It became a balancing act. I decided to be smart about my food consumption and if cutting something from my diet made me really sad, miserable, or any other negative emotion, I just wouldn't do it. You should all know by now how much I value quality of life over anything. Chocolate became part of that manifesto.

Now might be a good moment to mention that time I tried cannabis oil, the Rick Simpson oil to be precise. (Remember, at the time of writing this book, I've had this thing for eleven years and as such have had quite some time to try many, many things, with some successes and some epic fails.) In short: I got very high. Very paranoid. Thought I was going to kill Maren in her sleep. I then decided to stick it up my bum instead, as I read it gets to where it needs to be quicker without giving you the same side effects. That helped the paranoia and nausea, but as I lay on my bed, legs cocked, ready to insert a syringe into my arsehole, my cat Wilhelm glanced at me with a look that said *What the fuck are you doing?* Which was enough for me to not do it again.

Whenever I was doing well for a good amount of time, with minimal side effects and no drastic progression of the disease, I felt I'd become too passive in my approach to healing. I was really serious about having full control, so I always had some work to do before things started moving again – with incurable cancer there is at least one guarantee: that it *will* at some point start moving again. I started speaking to consultants in the area of integrative care. These were doctors who were not against conventional treatments but who very much focused on how the body could operate more effectively in order for those treatments to work to their best ability. My research led me to so many incredible experts, including an American naturopathic integrative oncologist and cancer survivor whom I still really admire today, Dr Nasha Winters. I've since read her book, listened to so many of her podcasts and even had the pleasure of meeting her once at my clever friend Sophie Trew's first ever cancer and holistic festival, called Trew Fields.

Dr Winters believes we must take a whole body, mind and spirit approach to cancer treatment. She doesn't believe cancer happens just because of genetic mutations or bad luck; it's instead a metabolic disorder that occurs in response to how we are feeding and treating our bodies and, therefore, our genomes. Through epigenetics (remember that clever word that may help us to understand why I got cancer and my twin didn't?) we may have the ability to influence gene expression and mitochondrial function through diet, lifestyle and thoughts. As she puts it, 'that's powerful medicine'. Our systems are disturbed because of modern life, and if we don't alter *how* we live, our bodies will never be healthy – oh and also, there's no such thing as a 'healthy' person before a cancer diagnosis, because this simply can't be true. I might have thought I was healthy in body, but I definitely wasn't in mind and spirit.

It's not enough to treat the tumour and cancer cells solely through aggressive strategies, which she does agree can and do work but more often than not at significant cost to the patient because conventional treatments damage healthy cells as well as cancer cells. Some treatments deplete the immune system, damage DNA, eradicate critical microbes in the gut, cause inflammation and oxidative stress, so it makes a lot of sense to make sure your body can cope with all that! What's more, and I think the most important thing of all and something I have concluded myself, is that she believes conventional treatment allows the patient to be passive: you get treatment and you wait for results. But there's a lot more you can do in the meantime that will ensure you don't become a victim, that you realise you have some control, too. It's ultimately about remembering that we are all unique – what's happened to us in our lives, what we've eaten, where we live (even race and socioeconomics and *many* health inequalities, if we're going to go there!) impacts what cancer we get and who gets it, but also all those things can impact our cancer-treatment outcome and, ultimately, our survival too (the sheer fact I am white means I am statistically more likely to survive Stage 4 breast cancer longer than my Black counterparts).

Because we are all unique (and maybe that was quite a long explanation to get me to my next point), you may be disappointed to hear that I won't be giving you a definitive answer on all the treatments I've tried and where I sourced all my information* (although I do *highly* recommend Dr Nasha Winters and people in that realm), because you are not me. My emotions are not your emotions, my background is not your background and add to that the very true and sad fact that my privilege might not be yours. Our systems are different, and to solidify Nasha's point about conventional treatment causing passivity, me giving you my personalised protocol would not only be unhelpful but perpetuate that issue too. Doing my own research, reading and reading, learning and learning, has helped me to make sense of my cancer a bit more; it has allowed me to feel like I *can* control certain aspects of my disease *and* it lets me decide (if my bank account allows!) what I will pursue in terms of integrative treatments and, ultimately, it's helped me accept my illness all the more. It has often made me think that I *could* eat/sleep/move to outsmart cancer, *but* it's a balance. I'm game to try things and I enjoy the exploration; I try to

---

* Also, with the ever-changing nature of my treatments my most up-to-date protocol would be out of date by the time you have this book in your hands. So instead you can find my complete and up-to-the-minute treatment (conventional and integrative) history on my website.

make an informed choice and, yes, there are probably a million more things I could add in, but I also want to live and not spend all my time either in the kitchen or in the bathroom (e.g. enemas) or worse, be totally broke. Cancer, in one way or another, comes with costs.

What I will pass on about about my treatments is that there's power derived from knowledge, that vegetables *really* do matter and that removing toxins from your life is the key – be that the food you eat, the chemicals in your household, the negative thoughts you think, or certain people. *And* it's possible to not compromise *all* your quality of life. Knowing there are *so* many options and avenues is OK. It's the self-assurance in the decision you've made that I think makes the biggest difference, and builds your bold nerve. Do the work, leave no room for doubt, but then surrender and have faith in your decision. That's what matters.

Lastly, healing never stops and that is actually *great*. We are conditioned to believe in, and want easily achieved gains, instant gratification and the ability to return to 'normal' after a burst of effort. But it doesn't work that way. The best thing you can hope for is a love affair with your healing journey. For it to be so fun, enjoyable and explorative that you don't even *want* to return to what once was. Cancer has shattered you, but also rebuilt you. That transformation might mean you do not fit in the same old conversations or relationships or thoughts or life any more. Maybe it really never has been about a cure; maybe what we should all be striving for is to be healed.

It's my hope that the longer I live, the more respect I build among the profession. I'm an outlier, someone who has survived cancer longer than average, and not just survived but manages to thrive. I think I knew I was one, not necessarily on the day I surpassed the average survival time of two to three years, but even before that. Outliers in geological terms are *young rock formations isolated among older rocks*. I see it as a metaphor. Sometimes I do feel like a young rock, trying to create a new path for anyone after me to step on to get across the river, while old approaches are creating a dam, a blockage. It's outliers that metaphorically rip up all the textbooks and theories and science. The more of us that speak up, the more minds might open.

The Year of the Sugar Cube

I can't go on. I'll go on.

Samuel Beckett

Until this moment I liked Russell Brand. A few years ago
I would have gone as far as to say I loved him; I even
owned his first book. But now as I lay in a tube, unable
to move, barely even allowed to breathe, or sigh, or
frown, or blink, he was annoying me. I'd not properly
considered whose voice or words I would have been able
to handle in that moment. I'd worked hard to put
together enough music – with the help of my friends Faye
and Jamie, who'd carefully selected songs for 'Kris's
Awesome Chill List' and 'Electro Chill for Kris', which
just about covered the first four hours of treatment – but
I needed to cram in a few more things and, thinking I'd
appreciate a podcast, in haste I'd added one with Russell.
As his highfalutin words slowly waltzed around my head,
I regretted my decision. He might have been saying

something deeply profound and brilliant, but I just felt annoyed. 'Let's try those breathing techniques,' I told myself. Maybe everything the oracle of breathing, friend and breath-technique expert Rebecca Dennis, had taught me would be useful now. Surely I could tap into all the stuff I'd learned, slow my breathing, drift off into a trance and maybe, just maybe, sleep?

It was wishful thinking. I was agitated. I was frustrated and I was scared. This was the second time I'd been in this tube, the second time two pins had to be screwed to my head that would be attached to a frame to keep my head as still as possible. They were treating more multiple, tiny, pretty harmless at current size, tumours that had sprouted in my brain. Just five months ago I had fifteen. They had all fully responded, in other words died from this very treatment, so we all knew this would work again. But it didn't make the experience any better.

I was lucky to be having this treatment at all. In January 2018, following my usual routine three-monthly scans, I got the news I wasn't exactly prepared for. It had been almost two years of a relatively breezy time on the drug palbociclib – except for the mouth ulcers. Now things had been moved up a gear. I was feeling particularly fit and strong, as I'd spent the previous month in Sri Lanka at an ayurvedic retreat doing daily Kundalini yoga and eating soul-nourishing food. In fact, I was almost convinced

Duncan would be telling me the cancer had fucked off completely. But nope. My current treatment had an average progression-free time of about eighteen months and that's exactly what I got out of it. I was disappointed. It was a drug that was hailed as one of the latest breakthroughs; why oh *why* could I not have eked out a bit more time with it? That thought was quickly sidelined, as the news of the brain tumours needed some attention.

'We can see about three, maybe four tiny lesions in your brain right now,' Duncan told me over the phone, our way of communicating now. The way I had decided was best for communicating. It avoided that horrendous wait in the Sunrise Centre. As I assumed and hoped, he told me I'd be getting the same treatment I'd received on my previous two brain tumours in 2012 and 2014, very targeted stereotactic treatment, only it would have to be done in Devon, as they didn't have the machines needed to do it in Cornwall. Fine. That was OK. I'd travelled for treatment before, so that would be fine. A rough plan was set. For the time being I could breathe just enough to get me through days without blind panic. I wouldn't be completely calm until a fixed date was pencilled and underlined three times in my Filofax (hey, come on now, even millennials like to have this stuff in writing).

I was in London when I expected to hear back with a firmer plan. I was, as per usual, darting between meetings and appointments. I was speed walking to my monthly mistletoe infusion on Wimpole Street when my phone buzzed. It was my CNS. Expecting her to simply confirm a date for treatment, she was instead calling to tell me that Derriford Hospital in Devon wouldn't be able to carry out my treatment because, on closer inspection – using what I imagined/understood was a device that allowed them to zoom in a few more pixels than the computers in Cornwall – they had discovered there were more like eleven tumours on my recent scan and thus I was outside their treatment bracket. They drew the line at ten. It was irrelevant that I was totally well – my doctor's notes said I had a performance score of 0, which, I found with the help of Google, meant I was functioning much like you. The scale ranges from 0 to 4, with 0 being fully functional and asymptomatic, and 4 being bedridden. It was irrelevant that I'd had super-targeted radiotherapy to two tumours before, that I had responded *very* well, and it had helped me live a pain-free, brain-tumour-free life for six bloody years. It was also, seemingly, according to my CNS, non-negotiable.

'So, as you know, the only option we have for treatment here in Cornwall is whole brain radiotherapy, so I'll need to get that booked in for you. When are you back in Cornwall?'

I had to stop her there. I was already very aware of what was on offer in Cornwall and I was also already very convinced I wouldn't be having that treatment, as there was absolutely no need. Let me explain this in layman's terms: picture a walnut, then a sledgehammer. You get me? Frying my ENTIRE brain, every last inch of it would, *yes*, of course zap the eleven (I mean, were they even sure it was eleven?) brain tumours, but also it would fry every inch of healthy cancer-free brain cell I owned. It would leave me possibly eternally hairless and maybe with cognitive issues FOR LIFE. Me. Kris Hallenga. Perfectly well, 'performing' well at o. Nah. No way.

'I need to discuss this with Duncan,' was my first reply, holding back the tears, to the CNS.

'OK, well, I'm not sure when he's free, but for now let me get you booked in for WBR.'

'That won't be necessary. I am not having that treatment. I need to speak to Duncan.' My voice was firm, but also on the verge of an almighty breakdown in the middle of a busy London street.

'OK, leave it with me.' Never have I ever left anything with anyone since that very day I was told I 'didn't have breast cancer'. This was no exception.

Breathless, clueless, motionless, I couldn't think of anything to do but call my friend Sophie. Yes, I could have phoned Maren or Mum or a London friend whose arms I could be in within thirty minutes, depending on current traffic and Tube service, but something was telling me that I needed a plan more than I needed hugs and tissues. Sophie was a Hodgkin lymphoma survivor, a health coach and had set up the UK's first cancer and holistic therapies festival called Trew Fields (it is more fun than it sounds, I promise!). And not just that: she was my wise owl, my oracle, and although she might not have a solution, she would undoubtedly have a way of making things OK.

'Sophie, they want me to fry my whole brain, but I'm not going to let them. I need another option: who should I speak to? What should I do? Who do I call? HELP ME!' I think I babbled.

'Kris, *breathe*,' she no doubt said. She was the calmest person, who could handle my reaction without unhelpful emotion.

'There will be another way. I will text Sophie now [another Sophie], who I know got targeted treatment – had to fight for it, mind, but got it privately. She will have contacts.'

Great. Of course, I did already know Sophie S had been in a similar boat – I knew the status of most outspoken outliers on the block – but that doesn't automatically mean you can just call them at the drop of a hat. But my hat was a heavy one, it had landed with a thud, and in that moment two Sophies said the words I needed to hear. Those two Sophies helped me walk to my mistletoe appointment. They had said enough encouraging stuff to let me get through the rest of the hours of that day.

I stumbled into the infusion clinic very blotchy-faced. I shared my recent news and predicament with a kind nurse whose job it was to find a vein and hook me up to a bag of mistletoe – something I'd started doing following a trip to a clinic in Scotland in spring 2016. After meeting the mistletoe god that is Dr Geider, and hearing him discuss immune-boosting mistletoe treatment and research at a conference, I decided, after more investigating, to undergo an intensive course at his clinic in Aberdeen and then followed it up with monthly infusions and twice-weekly injections ever since. It was proving to be a massive boost to my energy levels.

My head was in overdrive, trying to focus on Sophie's wise words about staying calm, reminding me that I'd jumped many hurdles before and that I'd get over this one too. She was, of course, right: I'd been in this very situation countless times, but it still felt alien; every time it felt like an untrodden path leading to heck knows where. I think it also had something to do with the fact that thoughts these days were louder. In Cornwall I had fewer distractions than when I was heading up the charity in London and living with friends. Now I had more time for feelings and worries to fester, but also more time to really allow them and work through them, too. Before long Sophie S was sending me helpful information about the treatment she'd managed to score privately; just knowing that someone else had fought to save their brain cells made me feel like less of a lunatic. It made me feel far less alone. But still I felt I needed to cast the net even wider I racked my brain for any and all contacts, my head working like one of those Rolodex business-card wheels, flicking from one person to another. Then I remembered the person who'd helped me think outside the box before – the consultant at Marie Curie Hospice in Hampstead, Dr Faye Gishen. She knew me and understood me more than most. I fired an email off to her and within the hour she replied, saying she was contacting someone urgently. Even now, writing this, I'm having to remind myself to breathe like I did that day. Those moments of intense stress and desperation apparently just don't leave you.

I'd arranged to meet my friend Fearne (she of TV presenting, book writing and Happy Place podcasting fame) at a café some days before the bad news, and now that day had arrived I was terrified to go because, to be honest, I'd never let her see this side of me before. Fearne bounded into my life in 2011, shortly after she'd taken part in a charity trek to Machu Picchu for another breast cancer charity. One of the other trekkers was Jenny (who'd sent me that email not long after CoppaFeel! was born). On sharing her story with Fearne, Jenny of course told Fearne all about how CoppaFeel! had been the reason she even pushed her doctors to investigate her breast cancer symptoms in the first place, and this chat and their friendship led to Fearne agreeing to do a half-marathon in aid of

CoppaFeel! The day I received an email from Fearne I knew she A) was a good egg and B) would be doing a hell of a lot more than running a half-marathon for us. She was my idea of a dream patron for the charity: fucking cool, young and sassy, honest, open, compassionate and a DOER. I remember first meeting her at an awards evening and coyly walking up to her to say hi, and she did what she has done since: listened, agreed to help, and saw that promise through. What started off as a relationship for CoppaFeel! soon blossomed into a true friendship for me, cemented with a shared love for cat-print clothing.

So until this moment I'd only ever seen Fearne when I was in a good place, when I had exciting plans to share, fun things to update her on, and on this day she got the complete opposite. I had no energy to mask my sadness and fear, but there was something about the way she held me that didn't make me even want to try. She allowed me to wallow, to cry, to talk it all out and barely eat the delicious food sitting in front of me. I soon learned that she could handle the hard conversations as well as the good. I spent the whole lunch date talking about myself and it was excruciating, but also so needed. It's only now that I am glad I shared a side of me that was as real as the confident charity CEO one Fearne had always met before. What's a friendship if you can't embrace each other's thrilling highs and earth-shattering lows?

*

By the end of the day Faye had emailed me the name of an NHS oncologist who specialises in primary and secondary brain tumours at University College London Hospitals. I would still need to do no end of chasing to ensure she got my latest images and knew what she was dealing with. You'd think this process would be easy, but it's not, and it involves emails and calls and pleading and begging for someone to send info about patients to another doctor. Sometimes this can take days; sometimes it takes months. I was exasperated by the time that week ended. I was staying with Simon, and needed a lot of cheering up with sushi and wine.

One week later the oncologist had reviewed my case; add another week to that and I found myself palm sweating in the waiting room at the Macmillan Cancer Centre near Euston with Maren. I wasn't sure what they'd be saying to me, but the fact they were seeing me at all filled me with enough hope and assurance that they'd think of something other than frying my entire healthy brain. I saw Dr Fersht, the consultant oncologist, and a brain surgeon called Mr Kitchen, along with a brilliant, kind, calm Irish CNS named Orla. My name was called and I walked into yet another consultation room, a new seating arrangement, and yet another new hospital, hoping to hear what I needed to hear: that I'd be treated according to my needs, with my quality of life considered, regardless of what the textbook or rulebook said. After the initial pleasantries and me explaining how I ended up there and my lengthy cancer history, they said my favourite few words of the English language: we can treat you. My shoulders lowered to a more reasonable level and my lungs filled with air.

'We will get you in for some very targeted gamma-knife therapy to treat the tumours we can currently see and anything that may be visible on the day.'

Gamma knife was pretty similar to the treatment I'd received to my pesky previous solo brain lesions, only it takes much longer, is a bit more intensive and requires very, *very* precise measurements and tumour targeting involving a head frame. It was the most amazing technology and I felt so lucky to get access to it.

'Fine. Yup. Sure. Anything,' I blurted, because really all I cared about in that moment was that they were prepared to spare my precious beautiful brain from unnecessary frying. Orla walked out of the room with us to ensure we understood what was about to happen next. I'd be booked in for treatment pretty smartish. I'd hear from them soon.

Three weeks later I received gamma-knife therapy to fifteen tiny pinhead-sized tumours, in total less than one cubic centimetre of my brain. Before leaving the clinic in Queen Square, London, where I was being treated, Dr Fersht came to see me and check how I got on. She was happy with how it all went and told me that on that day I had received one gray of radiation. I don't really need to explain to you what that exactly means, but what you do need to know is that receiving whole brain radiotherapy is thirty gray – essentially a heck of a lot more radiation than I needed. A treatment that, unlike gamma knife, cannot be repeated. It either works, with potentially detrimental side effects, or it doesn't. A treatment we could, much like the IV chemotherapy I was offered by Dr Hope, put on the shelf for an even rainier day. Dr Fersht was kind enough to give me the reassurance I so badly needed: that I'd made the right call. 'I'm glad you came to see us,' she said before leaving. I almost hugged her and maybe I would have if I didn't still have a frame bolted to my head. I sighed with relief.

And within five months I was back again. In the same neurology clinic in the basement of Queen Square, at an unreasonably early hour, about to have brand-new tumours zapped. You see, although the treatment was very targeted, killing any current active cancer spots and sparing all my healthy brain cells, it couldn't ensure new ones didn't sprout.

This time I knew the procedure, but knowing what was about to happen second time round was actually worse than the shock of the first time. I knew the pain of the injection to numb my skull; I knew the pressure of the screws being drilled into the front and back of my head. I knew the wait between frame fitting and actually being treated, while they planned my treatment, measured each tumour and worked out where exactly to send the cancer-destroying beams. I was familiar with the guessing game of how long I might be in the tube for this time and I knew the faces of the other patients who were either waiting, like me, or were just being wheeled out of the treatment in a wheelchair (even though I could walk, they insist on a wheelchair while you're wearing the metal frame attached to your head in case you trip and, well, I don't need to explain the rest. Still, I hate wheelchairs: they make me feel like a sick person).

Not sure that even if you tried that you'd guess six hours. It took six hours (including a wee break and a cry break) for me to have all the tiny active tumours treated, which, in the end, were around twenty. I never bothered to ask what the exact number was; it was already horrific enough to know it had jumped up from six, when I initially got my scan results, just three weeks before.

I would go on to have this treatment for the third time just four months later (with the help of some mild sedatives) following another routine scan that showed my head was glowing with yet more tiny glow-worm beasts. In total the fifty-seven tiny tumours I had zapped with gamma-knife therapy in 2018 fitted inside a sugar cube.

When you put it like that, it seems so harmless, right? What harm could something the size of a sugar cube do? Well, nothing, of course. Cancer cannot kill you until it finds a way to overwhelm your entire system. I just needed to find a way to keep blocking it. I needed constant roadblocks – like the ones on the A303 you don't know about until you hit them late in the evening, adding at least two hours on to your journey time (if you know, you know). I needed something equally annoying and tedious for cancer.

I was more than aware that my systemic treatment needed a rethink. Whatever I was doing clearly wasn't quite enough. Cancer was finding a new, clever way to get past all my new-found techniques. Once again – despite the constant fear and heartache, and the nuisance of having to be driven around everywhere, as I was not allowed behind the wheel – I gained a new level of respect for this disease. How it managed to outsmart everything and find a new way to gain energy and fuel to grow blew my mind.

After yet more days of researching, deliberating and a very painful liver biopsy to do a genome test to discover what treatments would be effective, if any, the year of the sugar cube ended with me starting a new systemic treatment, an oral chemotherapy called capecitabine, alongside my by now pretty extensive non-NHS treatments. At the time of writing this book, I have been on this combination for two years with no new brain tumours, very few side effects and a truckload of renewed hope.

Breathe

Don't know about you, but I just needed to remind myself to breathe. That's all.

Worthiness

I am deserving of a full, long life like you, like anyone.

I am a pretty open book when it comes to my cancer diagnosis (I mean, here you are reading an entire book about it). I see it as an opportunity to teach others how to live with cancer, despite it and in spite of it. This leaves me sometimes pretty vulnerable and exposed, especially online. In being more open and honest in sharing my life, I allow for opinions, thoughts, suggestions. I welcome them all, but I don't necessarily let them all flood my consciousness. I guess you call that a healthy boundary. What I find most hard to grapple with is the contrast in responses I get from sharing suffering and joy. How I will get a bigger response when I'm hurting than when I'm simply living. I think we're conditioned to judge and pit ourselves against each other – especially as women. We feel like we need to downplay our strengths to avoid threatening anyone. We find it easier to rally around someone who is in pain than someone who is standing tall. The same issue is apparent in charities too. Charities need to show struggle and headlines need to be sensationalised for people to help and support, instead of, ya know, boosting them when they're flying and changing or saving lives.

Standing on a stage speaking to hundreds of people, I feel strong. I feel powerful. I feel liked. I feel like I'm allowed to be me. But is that because I've been given a pass because of cancer? Sometimes I think cancer patients are given a ticket to live unapologetically and to love ourselves when we exist in a world that insists we have no right to. Would I be cheered from the sidelines quite so much without a deadly illness? That's something I think about a lot. Would you like me and admire me and *see* me without cancer? Without it I think I'd be plagued by fear of judgement. Society and our culture teaches us (womenfolk) to be self-doubting, reserved and to apologise for everything. I have to almost use cancer as an excuse for my worthiness, that I am little without it. But that surely can't be true? That is surely something I have learned through social media or just life. Something has shat on my worthiness. We're more proud of people who achieve through pain and suffering than those who are just being unapologetically loud and proud and brilliant and wise and give no fucks. *Why?*

Too often I receive messages from women detailing their terminal cancer diagnosis. How they feel like they've been given up on, how they don't know how to cope, how they need help in knowing what treatment to choose, and more often than not it will end with 'and I have an X-year-old that I need to stay alive for'. I don't doubt and can't even comprehend the pain of leaving a child, but sometimes I wonder if that woman *truly* knows that *she* is enough to stay alive for and that *she* was worthy enough of a response from me (if I have the brain power and capacity to give one, that is) without the child detail. And how do you think it makes me and other non-mums feel when time and time again I read an article about someone with a terminal illness and always, always it must mention they have a young child. The story is sad enough, the struggle is real enough, without anything or anyone added to it. In needing to share that this person is someone's mother, someone's daughter, someone's sister, we are conditioned to think we're not enough to simply be *someone*.

Let me hear you say this out loud (or in your head is cool too):

I am worthy of surviving cancer (or substitute with any brand of turd if not applicable).

I am worthy of hope.

I am worthy of success, joy, love and laughter, with or without offspring. With or without cancer.

PS. Support charities even when they're not crying for help.

A Strong Reason for Living

If there was a moment, just one moment, that I stayed alive for through all those years of scans and results and treatments, it was 16 May 2015, when I walked Maren down a very sandy aisle on a beach in Cornwall. I thought then, *If this is the one thing I have been granted to stay alive for, and if, like in the fairy tales, the clock strikes twelve and my time is up after this, then that would be OK.* Life couldn't get much fuller than this, could it? And if it could, I wasn't even that bothered to find out for sure. Because in that instant I understood what being alive meant.

I had even played a bargaining game in my head: *Kris, would you give this up, being here, at your twin sister's wedding, if it meant you didn't have cancer any more?* My answer was a decisive no. I wondered if I'd have felt this gushy if I hadn't had cancer for the past six years, and if Maren and I hadn't been through some of the hardest days of our lives together, or if the silent but deadly threat that I might not live to see them marry hadn't been hanging over us from the second she announced she was engaged. If I had ever been anywhere near 'grateful' for having cancer, this would be the time. I was grateful that this all mattered so very much. Cancer slapped gratitude in my face and hit me around the chops repeatedly. Huge spotlights are shone on occasions in your life with cancer, and this was one of those times, and, bugger me, it was blindingly bright. I think it was that moment with Maren when time stood still and I realised everything was enough. Perhaps there had been times before this day when I had been close to that epiphany too, but for some reason that slow walk in the sunshine, sand between the toes, with Mar, crystallised it; that first dance with me, her and Graham, recreating the famous *Romy and Michele's High School Reunion* dance cemented it (yes, we peaked).

Although I don't like to plan far ahead in case I don't live to see something happen, I will, when big things are on the horizon, imagine with every fibre of my being that I will be there. When I commit to an event unnervingly far in the future I am putting some faith in believing that I have a future. I do this sparingly and consciously because I try, as much as I can, to be present and happy with what is and has been without wishing for more. Call it self-preservation, call it what you want – it works for me. I don't promise, I don't overcommit, but somewhere deep inside I sometimes allow myself to believe in a strong possibility that I will still be alive to witness something and be part of something special. I allow myself to breathe in that air of possibility (that same air, remember, that my doctor, Mr Dawson, all those years ago, allowed to circulate in the room the day he told me I had incurable cancer).

When Maren told me G had proposed, I was standing in busy Charles de Gaulle Airport waiting for a flight to London. I had a feeling as soon as I saw her FaceTime call flash up on my phone that she was about to tell me something significant. They were spending time together on the Isles of Scilly; it was cute; conditions were perfect. It hadn't been a strong inkling, not as strong as I had hoped and imagined from, ya know, my childhood delusions and *The Parent Trap*, but it was a jolt of something, for sure. We were as teary and snotty as you can imagine as she showed me the pretty ring Graham had had made for her. My head quickly jumped ahead to planning her hen do (which, can I just say, was a masterpiece, including the bit where we had a professional choreographer teach us the *Flashdance* dance, which they filmed and turned into a music video) and from there it jumped to the wedding and then next thing I knew I wasn't just mentally there, I was physically, every last fibre of me, *there*. And after that I could settle into feeling like everything beyond that point was a bonus.

*

Talking of bonuses, if you'd told me some years ago I'd witness the birth of my first nephew, I'd have firstly laughed in your face but then secondly shrugged and said 'perhaps' while secretly hoping beyond hopes that I *would* indeed see that day and live that experience with Maren. Fast-forward four years from the wedding. Little did I know that seeing the birth of Herbie Ray William Sheldon wouldn't just be confirmation of a reason to stay alive, but it would give me an entirely new meaning of life and love. Add to that a whole new appreciation for the human body, women's bodies, and for Maren. It took for her to scream in agony one inch from my face to understand just a tiny percentage of the struggle she felt in watching me go through the pain of cancer. Of course, this was a different kind of pain, one that produced wonderful life, but nonetheless I felt as helpless, as fearful, as dumbfounded, as speechless as I'm sure, and know, she has felt at some point over these past eleven years.

That moment Herbie flopped out and into the birthing pool, was fished out by the midwife and handed to Mar, and her eyes went from her screaming newborn to me, was when I saw in them something that solidified a trusted, unforsaken bond that will live on, whether we are both alive or not. When I held Herbie and breathed in all his magnificence (while Maren was having her bits sewn back up), he confirmed something very reassuring that I sort of already knew: that life goes on. 'Kris, I've got this,' I read in his eyes. Young Kris who thought she'd pursue happiness without really knowing what that meant is a little clearer on that meaning now.

One of my oracles (in other words, author of a book I devoured and will happily harp on about to anyone who will listen), Dr Kelly Turner, has spent many years analysing the similarities between the lives of people like me, the ones who defy the statistics and, in her words, reach 'radical remission'. She couldn't work out why we had never been studied before, how there was never much emphasis on *why* people sometimes live much longer than others. I guess the most cynical answer to that would be that there's no way of objectively concluding such a study without a GINORMOUS cohort and huge investment, and without guarantee of anything replicable and useful for future cancer patients, nothing you could reproduce in a lab, patent and put a price on. But as Gabor Maté says:

Not all essential information can be confirmed in the laboratory or by statistical analysis. Not all aspects of illness can be reduced to facts verified by double-blind studies and by the strictest scientific techniques. We confine ourselves to a narrow realm indeed if we exclude from accepted knowledge the contribution of human experience and insight.

Undeterred, she investigated and dug deep for correlations anyway. She defines radical remission as someone whose cancer has gone away without using any conventional medicine; or a cancer patient who tries conventional medicine, does not go into remission, then switches to alternative methods of healing, which *do* lead to remission; or a cancer patient who uses conventional medicine and alternative healing methods at the same time in order to outlive a statistically dire prognosis (i.e. any cancer with a less than 25 per cent chance of five-year survival). When I casually picked Dr Turner's book to read during the retreat in Sri Lanka, I never identified myself as someone in remission, I just thought it looked like an interesting read, until I ingested her definition and realised the book was very much speaking to me. I remember looking up from the book and reading the definitions out loud to my friend Kay for some sort of confirmation that I did qualify for the last point. Dr Turner had discovered nine similarities between the many cancer patients to whom she spoke in depth, which she has since upgraded to ten for her latest book, *Radical Hope*. I'm not sure if this will be a surprise to you or not, but most of the similarities aren't physical, they are mental. They are to do with mindset.

It would be easy to say that each outlier was simply lucky and that the similarities were coincidental, but to put *my* experience purely down to luck is, for me, almost offensive. In defying the odds this long I have come to recognise the work I've put in. That's not to say anyone who doesn't live beyond the textbook average never tried 'hard enough' or did anything 'wrong'; it's more an acknowledgment that *some* consciousness has gone into *me* still being here (and *yes*, maybe I want a pat on the back from time to time), as well as a lot of stuff I wasn't aware of. One of the ten aspects is one she simply calls 'having strong reasons for living'. Now this might seem a pretty obvious one and something you'd assume most people would align with after a cancer diagnosis. But it's not enough to not want to die; it's about letting go of all fear and living most authentically, unapologetically and vividly. As she says, 'Having strong reasons for living means focusing on why you want to keep living instead of the fact that you might die sooner than you had hoped.' What she saw in the radical remission case studies wasn't necessarily 'a complete fearlessness about death but rather enough desire for life that their fear of death does not become all-encompassing'.

In combination with the nine other key factors, which are: exercise, spiritual connection, empowerment, increasing positive emotions, following your intuition, releasing suppressed emotion, changing your diet, using herbs and supplements, and increasing social support, this desire to live completes the package. To be clear, they are hypotheses, not facts, but ones that do no harm to live by, regardless of cancer. A positive mindset is not a standalone cure for cancer, and its toxic overuse and over-prescription to cancer patients in society is frankly annoying and trite. And as the novelist Matt Haig so brilliantly put it in a tweet on Twitter: 'Positive thinking is not positive thinking if it allows no negativity. Expecting life to be a wholly positive experience will only lead to more suffering. Seeing the connection between joy and despair, seeing the entirety of experience within a single moment is the way forward.' *This* dollop of wisdom in symphony with access to the best possible drugs, the best possible nutrients, physical activity and more, can work in your favour; it definitely has in mine. I'm under no illusion about my situation, but to be limited by it isn't an option either. Plus, positivity can't protect us from all sources of external uncontrollable stresses like, for example, a shoddy government and the destruction of our beautiful world (I could go on) and we NEED to be MOVED by these stressors to enable action.

You'll have seen throughout this book that in one way or another I have embraced many of the factors from Dr Turner's list. Whether they are the reason I am still alive today or not is actually irrelevant though. I think what has become very clear to me is that how I got here stretches way beyond any theories, scientific or otherwise. What started as a dodgy cell gone wrong somewhere along the line in my life turned into a lesson I didn't know I needed. A lesson of self-discovery, self-compassion

and self-belief. It's only in writing this book that I truly understood that cancer gave huge meaning to the before-cancer Kris and continues to give meaning to the with-cancer Kris and the Kris that exists today. In writing this book I have honoured the little symbiosis created between me and cancer – it's only in looking back at the past that I can finally permit the past to become past.

Who I am today, as I write this, is the sum of twenty-three years of self-doubt + a cancer diagnosis + eleven years of learning and discovering who I really am. And I like who I am. I've realised what the real turd and what the real glitter is in all of this. Of course, starting a charity that has helped many people licked many of my wounds, it helped me realise my skills, passion and talent, but it would be cancer that provided the biggest sparkle of all. Cancer became my way out, not CoppaFeel!. The turd – or I should say turds, plural – were the ugly, detrimental thoughts in my head; cancer and everything that followed was the glitter. CoppaFeel! elevated me, and healed parts of me cancer could never reach, but without the disease I'd never have been saved from the wreckage. It has allowed me to take up space on this planet. It's given me confidence, pride, a swagger that without cancer you would probably look at with disdain (it's cool, it's not your fault – you were trained not to trust women who are smashing the shit out of life).

Cancer gave me permission to stop accepting everyone

else's thoughts, feelings, behaviours and start a line of communication with what I really wanted, and who I wanted to be in this world. CoppaFeel! helped me to gain my voice. I needed a label to hang my existence on – survivor, fighter, warrior but now that I've found myself I can shed that safety blanket. I am fully able to exist without needing to say that I HAVE CANCER (I don't need the worship that these words produce) and I AM A CEO OF A CHARITY because I was and am enough without the clout. I am enough without anyone's validation. Wow. I want us to find our superpowers, our strengths, our BIG-ness, our glitter without a terminal illness, and discover and relish our reasons for living. Please do that for me. I am giving you permission to exist fully without cancer. Without turds. Just the glitter.

In Summary: Not Dead

Dear twenty-three-year-old Kris,

My girl, you are at the foothills of something really rather shite. But you already know that, so I am here to tell you all the things that are good about your diagnosis – I know that sounds utterly ridiculous to you right now, but stay with me. You are frightened, of course you are, but in the darkest of moments I want you to remember one thing: life will go on in the most spectacular of ways. I need you to hold on; I need you to accept that life will drastically change and although you fear change so much, it will all – I mean mostly – be good. Uncertainty is so scary, we know that, but it will make you seize many opportunities and by that I mean MANY glorious 'fuck it' moments.

You don't know this right now, but you have all the strength you need to survive cancer, its treatments and side effects, and you will actually be glad when they finally remove your boob later this year. You will choose not to have reconstruction. Some years later you will decide to have the other boob removed too, not because you have to but because you want to. You look KILLER in a low-cut V top.

You know how, during the last two years, you have had a strange relationship with your body – trying to be slimmer, not really knowing why – well, guess what, sister, you are leaving that shit behind you. Along with the boy you currently love and feel so betrayed by – he will fade from your mind, TRUST ME, he will. But you know that thing he said about how HE caused your cancer? Perhaps there's something in it.

Talking of love, it will play a huge role in your survival, but not love with anyone, just with yourself. You know how Niall told you that you beat the odds getting cancer at this age so you'd beat the odds surviving it? He is right. You see, I know you will find this very hard to believe, but you will still be alive in eleven years' time. I repeat: YOU WILL STILL BE ALIVE IN ELEVEN YEARS' TIME. Take that in. The reason you find this hard to believe is because you haven't heard of anyone who has survived this long, have you? And when you stupidly googled mortality rates the other night, you thought two to three years was the average and the norm. But you are not the norm. You know how, despite this statistic, you somehow, weirdly, knew you were going to be OK? Well, you will be more than that. You will no longer need to see proof that people live with cancer for a long time because you become the proof.

Although you may not feel like it on many days, you will get up, have a shower, brush your hair, do your make-up, put the kettle on and get on with your day. This will sometimes feel like the biggest achievement of the day, and that is OK.

It won't be long before you become someone with a purpose, an actual real-life reason to live, Kris! In fact, it will be just days before you lose all your hair to chemotherapy – and by the way, you have a great head and many people will tell you this. That will, at times, get annoying. Oh, and also you will proclaim that because you've lost your hair you will never complain about a bad hairdo again. This is bullshit. You will have many of those. And you will complain.

Although Mr Dawson just advised that you probably shouldn't be jumping out of a plane any time soon because you have a cancerous tumour on your spine, you will at some point run a 10k and then a half-marathon. I can't explain this phenomenon, and to be honest you won't enjoy these events, but you will turn into quite the stubborn bitch in an effort to prove that you simply 'can', which is useful because when it comes to cancer the focus too often is on stuff you can't do. And although you don't enjoy running, you will rope countless friends and then hundreds of strangers into running for your charity.

Yes, I said charity. It will be called CoppaFeel! – you will come up with that name and your friends will think it's a good one, but you won't be entirely sure whether they are just being nice because you have cancer. But it sticks. Sounds like a lot of hard work, doesn't it? Well, it will be, especially as you choose to do it when the economy is on its arse. But as the writer Glennon Doyle says (in a few years' time), it's the 'right kind of hard', a type of hard that pays back tenfold. It will also be the best thing you will ever decide to do and maybe even be one of the reasons you survive for as long as you do. Although of that I can't be sure.

What I can be sure of is that CoppaFeel! will change the lives of many people. Not long from now you will hear from people who have been diagnosed early because of what you do. And then those messages will become a regular thing.

You will make a good boss. A boss of the charity and a boss of your own health. There is not a straight path to healing. You will have to take the reins and navigate your way through the medical system and jump through many hoops. It will be frustrating, frightening and you will find yourself in the loneliest of places, but with the help of so many incredible people you will carry on. You won't always know why, but you'll keep going.

You will realise you're a doer, not a planner, which may infuriate your staff, but you learn to appreciate people's unique ways of working and love them for it.

In the midst of chemotherapy you will meet a guy. The relationship will be blissful, sad, comforting and then a bit shit. So you break up. And you will possibly cry more than you did when your dad died and more than you did last night. Annoyingly, cancer doesn't give you a cloak that protects you from heartache. You are no less a human because you are facing something seemingly way larger and more life-threatening than any relationship could be.

You will shift your thinking. Instead of wanting someone to complete you, you will strive to live a life that others want to be part of. You will make your life so attractive for you that others might not resist it. You will ask yourself: How can I make myself such a fascinating companion for myself? So much so that you don't notice that no one is with you. At the same time, you will also decide that anyone who says they love being single because they can spread out in their double bed is lying.

After eight years of singledom, commitment will start to feel alien. So much so that you will be astounded when your garden perennials re-emerge each year. That doesn't mean you're not open to the idea that someone could slot into your life; it's just that you will not attach as much importance to it happening, and you won't need it to make you feel like you're really living.

You will dance sober a lot.

You'll have a much healthier relationship with food.
FOOD IS FUCKING GREAT.

You won't have a baby, but then we both know that children can be arseholes. I'm sorry to say that in eleven years' time you will still feel like you need to push this point about not actually wanting children. It will still not be a widely accepted phenomenon that a woman might really, truly not want to reproduce. BUT you will marvel at your friends for pushing babies out of their vaginas while you own two legendary cats.

You won't own a house (they don't give terminally ill people mortgages which is actually a bit shit).

You won't get married.

There won't be a cure.

Life will take on a whole new meaning. You will move to London and then to Cornwall because you will understand what you really want out of life.

You will make questionable fashion choices. Some things don't change.

You will experience pain, so much pain. Tramadol doesn't help you with that.

You will hide your fear under a mask of positivity.

You will accept death.

You'll make some monumental errors in your judgement of people.

You will at first get pissed off when people send you

unsolicited advice about various treatments you could try that you've not heard of, but then you will start to realise it comes from a good place and, whatever it is they are suggesting MIGHT actually be useful. Dismissing it is not very prudent and a bit rude.

You will have a godson named after you.

You will have a Neighbours-*themed thirtieth birthday party (you will be Charlene, of course). Mar will be Dee back from the dead. (Who knew you had such great ideas?)*

You will go to Disneyland Paris with a blue badge enabling you and your pals to skip ALL the queues.

You will watch sunrise in a crater in Hawaii.

Talking of travelling, you will go to Japan, Thailand, New York, Canada, Austria, Italy, Portugal, California, Iceland.

You will allow yourself to be vulnerable.

You will realise that there are forever some familiar constants throughout your life that the cancer cannot touch, such as:

- Your need to eat dessert with a small spoon.
- Your capacity to love and be loved.
- Your ability to blush easily.
- Your aptitude for finding the best gelato places.
- Your annoying nail-biting habit.
- Your love for dresses with pockets.

You will realise that you never have been, and never will be, a burden.

You will nearly shit yourself on BBC Breakfast, *and not in the metaphorical sense.*

Cancer won't be the first and last thought of your every day.

You will watch Mar give birth. Man, if you think cancer is gnarly, you will get quite the shock. The only reason you will be brave enough to be there is because you know you'll never be facing that yourself; you want to know what it's like so that when you are inevitably surrounded by parents you feel a little less like a loser outsider.

You will return to Australia as an adult and this time you will eat food consisting of more than three ingredients/not in the Woolworths reduced section.

Your name will be on an IMDB *page from playing yourself in a film.*

You will mastermind a collaboration with skate brand Vans and sell shoes GLOBALLY *in aid of CoppaFeel!*

You will see wonder in the mundane.

You will be so proud of the CoppaFeel! team (a fierce group of seventeen women!) that you might, at times, feel like bursting.

You will learn to love running into the cold sea. I'M NOT EVEN MAKING THIS SHIT UP.

Some days you won't feel like getting out of bed, so you don't.

You will be awarded an honorary doctorate in public administration – LOL, ain't that ridiculous?

You know how you dreamed of getting boob-check reminder labels into bras that day sitting around Mum's dining table? That'll happen.

You will hijack Page Three of the Sun and educate people to check their boobs.

The UK will vote to leave the EU. I know, I know, let's not get into that right now . . .

This thing called Instagram is about to be invented in which you share many pictures of your life. It will become sort of addictive, but some days your followers will keep you from drowning in sorrow and self-pity.

You will get cancer on the school curriculum. You think I am fibbing, but I am not.

You will say NO a lot.

You will say YES and accept help from friends, even though a little piece of you dies inside. Talking of friends, you have some bloody great ones. Some will come and go. And that's OK. You will love watching your friends live their lives. As one of your not-yet-but-soon-to-be favourite authors, Dolly Alderton, says, you can be moved by something and not need it for yourself. You will make many new mates and – this may sound

very strange – you may just thank cancer for them.
Especially one dressed in a cow outfit.

The death of your dad taught you so much about life
and its fragility, but it will hit you even harder when
some of the best people you have met die.

A music festival you organise that started off in a
small pub will grow to a point where you will not
recognise most of the people attending.

Not only will you move to Cornwall to be near
Maren, but you will realise your joint dream to make
cakes and sell coffees from a vintage truck you name
Beyoncé. You will give her this name because you
bought it when the real-life icon Beyoncé was expecting
twins. That makes sense to you.

You will celebrate your tenth cancerversary with all
the people you adore, wearing a cat costume, in the
Mediterranean biome at the Eden Project.

Eleven years living with cancer won't make the
uncertainty and fear disappear, but you will learn so
many ways of coping.

There will come a day when you look at your
predicament with great respect for you. In being more
appreciative of how you have coped, and continue to
cope, you'll gain acceptance. In its definition, acceptance
is 'the action of consenting to receive or undertake
something offered'. You were not offered cancer, but you
were offered an opportunity to learn SO **much** from

having it. It means you can accept it and all the lessons it's taught you and the life you've shaped around it. In doing so you accept that life is fleeting; you accept that cancer is, more than likely, going to kill you; you accept that life is a bit shit but around the prickly edges of shit it is also bloody magnificent. Acceptance is not weakness or a sign of giving in or giving up. It's many miles from that. Acceptance actually allows for control. In accepting your illness you start to let go of so much and just be. In accepting your fate you give yourself space and room to LIVE.

You will write a book in which you pen this letter because you know what a difference it would have made to you on that awful day when you found out your cancer was incurable. And maybe another frightened girl who is the same position as you will read it and sleep just that little bit easier tonight.

Kris, life goes on, and while living eleven years is so hard to comprehend, just believe in endless possibilities. You will look back over a decade in wonder and amazement and realise how far you have come. While I can't promise a life beyond that, I can assure you that life will already feel more than complete.

PS. 2020 is a shitshow. Don't ask.

Afterword

I ask you not to google whether I'm still alive. When you read this book it is possible that I'm no longer here. When I died or, in fact, how I died is irrelevant. In a rush to find out whether I'm gone you'd be undoing all the hard work I put into convincing you that what matters is how and why I lived. If you're going to be rushing to do anything after reading this book, it should be only this: to glitter your own turd. Oh, and also check your boobs.

To keep following my adventures, and for a complete history of my cancer treatments, head to my website howtoglitteraturd.com. For the full lowdown on checking your boobs/pecs/chest, head to coppafeel.org

Acknowledgements

It would have been nice if someone had warned me that book writing is essentially staring at a laptop screen for hours and hours saying the words, 'You are shit – how did you think you could write a book?' over and over, on repeat. So, it's a good job YOU, the reader, made all the internal anguish worthwhile. You have been guiding and willing me on more than you could ever know.

I have deliberated over the rest of this acknowledge-ment section for so long. I have left it to the very last minute to write because I just wasn't sure how my grati-tude for the people I am about to name would ever be truly, fully and meaningfully conveyed. But I am going to give it my best shot anyway (mainly because my editor really does want this in ASAP, sorry Imogen).

The trauma of my diagnosis runs deep. But in writing about it I have given it some space to air out. If I am truly honest, I am not sure I have written *everything* because perhaps some things are just too hard, but I would like to think that the words I have managed to force out of myself have appeased and soothed the ones I couldn't. Call it a writer's prerogative or maybe just a survival tactic. What I do know for sure, is that without the wonderful people in my life I would never have gone to the edge and been brave enough to take a leap and get this thing done. I really didn't realise the incredible cheerleaders I had in my life until now – although, cancer did give me a pretty good idea.

First off, Mar. (If you think I am crying at this point you would be correct.) My kettle-putter-onner, my lie detector, my perspective bringer, my eternal better half. You know it's not an exaggeration when I say that A) I would not still be here without you and B) without your belief in this book, I would never have even opened Word on my Mac to start it. Maybe if I was half the non-procrastinator you are, this thing might have been written some years ago, but your darn-right bossiness really has made this thing come to life. Mar, you've helped me broaden the depth and breadth of my appreciation for living. Thanks also for bringing G, Rambo and Herbie into my life. I love you all so much.

Mum! It's been twelve years and I have still not got closer to really truly knowing and understanding how hard it was for you to hear I had cancer, but then to be so strong and so stoic, so quickly and unrelentingly. You have put your everything on the line for me, Mar and Maike from the day each of us entered your womb and I am so glad I had such an incredibly indestructible woman to look up to.

Maike, my little big sis. I know your support for me, whether you are near or far, is unwavering. And I am always grateful for that.

Rosemary. The universe ensured you were with us on my worst day imaginable and you knew exactly what to do, namely to fill our bellies with delicious food when that task was so far from our minds. I am glad you stuck around long enough to teach me how to knit a scarf.

Hannah, my literary agent. Your patience and enthusiasm for this book NEVER FALTERED and I am SO happy we finally made it happen. Thank you for never giving up on me and sorry it took so long BUT YAY LOOK WE MADE A BOOK HAPPEN!!!!

Joelle. Thanks for reaching out to me not once, but twice and then taking me on at Unbound.

My Unbound editing team, Martha, Imogen, Victoria Millar, Kate Quarry and Hayley Shepherd, for helping to make my many thoughts and words make some sense. Thanks also to Anna Morrison for the epic cover design.

Elijah. Thanks for giving me the best advice anyone could which was simply to 'write'. (Kristian, seeing as you are my godson and namesake you deserve some kudos too. Thanks for growing up to be such a bloody good kid like your twin and special big up to your mama.)

Niall. I'm glad that you were right, even when I found

it so hard to believe at times. I'm also glad you came to check on me when I wasn't sure if I was actually OK.

Lou. Thanks for taking the rap for the blood-stained sheets at Adam's house by telling him it was your puke. That's friendship I didn't know I was lucky enough to have.

Mr Dawson, thank you for letting me believe that anything was possible.

Helen and Becky Measures, you women gave me that initial spark to get CoppaFeel! off the ground and I will (along with the many lives that have been saved) truly always be thankful.

My CoppaFeel! birthing partners who sat around Mum's table that monumental day: Lou, Ben, Rach, Mar, Adam and Hugo. And the many legends that hopped aboard thereafter, including Sarah, Liam, Bianca, Dave, Ed, James, Anna, Nicky, Dan, Makeda, Mary, Kirsten, Louis and Arthur.

Jamie. It takes a special person to dedicate SO much time and SO much energy to a mere idea. CoppaFeel! would hands down not be the success it is without you. Thank you for being part of this story from the beginning and for never bowing out, even when things got really fucking hard. You're the most talented marketeer I know and one of the best friends a girl with a shitty illness could have.

Hugo. Thanks for putting up with my many demands and tweaks and changes and ideas for our branding. And the muffins in the post. Still one of the kindest things anyone has ever done for me.

The Beach Break Live team. Thanks for not laughing at our bizarre request to come and chat about boobs with all your festival goers. I'm still not really sure you are aware just what you helped us kick-start, but I hope this book helps.

Erica. Thankful you were plonked into my life to quell those early chemo side-effect panics and fears and for making a dancefloor a lot more silly and fun.

Jane and the CRUK team. Thank you for giving me a voice and letting me share my story in the very early days when I was probably still baffled by it myself.

Phil Packer. A bow to you, for all your efforts to help young people and in fact anyone.

Peter Drummond. I am not sure you knew what you were letting yourself in for by allowing Maren, Dom and me to take over BDP Towers, but you gave us a base, a hub, a hive that helped us grow so quickly and efficiently. Also, Paul Hobbs, for not being too grumpy about the eye-watering amount of printing and posting we did.

Kate Lee. My heroine, my mentor, my friend. Goddammit woman, we need to clone you and make you CEO of all charities the world over. World problems would be solved a hell of a lot quicker.

Jenny. Your email made it all make sense. Thank you.

Steve Stretton. As exhausting as it is to be in a meeting

with you, your passion and support in making the coolest and most innovative campaigns come to life is remarkable. We love you.

Faye Gishen. Thank you for coming into my life when I needed to regain trust in myself, my body and my mind.

Emily. I know there is a part of you that gets such a kick out of finding a vein in my hand or foot, even after many laborious failed attempts. Thank you for helping me take back some control.

Duncan. You helped me regain confidence in a medical team and understand the importance of quality of life. I'm lucky to have found you. PS. Hurry up and find a cure.

Sophie Trew. My oracle in times of need and times of tequila and spirulina. What would I, and a million other cancer peeps, do without you??

Sophie Sabbage. It takes a hope-bringer to know a hope-bringer. Thanks for holding out a hand during despair and thank you for teaching me it's possible to RIP before I die.

Lucy Kalanithi. Thank you for allowing me to use your late husband's incredibly wise words in this book.

Claire. Trustee meetings would be a hell of a lot less fun without you and your love of fizz. I'm so glad you had a cool job title that led me to you.

Team Boobs. YOU GUYS. Thank you for keeping the flame lit, for cradling my legacy and for giving a shit every, single, day. I am so endlessly proud of everything we achieve as a boss team.

Dom. I don't envy the task you took on in working for me and Maren at the very beginning, but I am so glad you did it, undeterred.

Hen. Pro tea drinker and mother hen. Only you could break awful financial news to me and still make me feel it would all be OK.

Nat. You took on one heck of a job and I am so grateful and proud, always.

All our trustees, past and present. Thank you for the guidance.

All the friends I made over boob chats and face painting in a festival field, thanks for lifting my spirits.

Fluorescent PR crew, I've never known commitment and hard work like it. Forever grateful.

Aya, my sweet friend. I never wanted you to know what any of this actually felt like IRL, but then again, I never doubted that you could take it all on so effing brilliantly. Eternally grateful that two douchebags brought us together.

Boobettes. MY BOSS BITCHES, I salute you, I love you.

Fearne, Gi, Dawn and Annie. I am so honoured you all read my book before anyone else and that you gave it such incredible reviews and shared so many wonderful words with me. You have NO IDEA how shit-scared and then relieved I was. Thank you.

Georgette. There are not many people who could drag me out of a very sad and hopeless hole. Well done for having that ability. And for 'plodding along' with me.

Samia. How lucky I am to have learned so much from, and to have been guided by you.

Rebecca Dennis. Thank you for teaching me the power of breath.

Dr Geider and Barbara, my mistletoe dream team. Thank you.

Neil, Matt and October Films. Never not proud of our film and the many, MANY lives it has impacted.

Dr Kelly Turner, for reminding me of the power of hope.

The researchers in the labs creating the drugs that keep me here.

Stace. Thanks to you none of this stuff ever went to my head. What a knob I might be without you.

Simon. I think you have witnessed most of my tears and fears and yet still found a way to make me laugh and then subsequently fed me sushi. That takes some skill. And I love you for that.

Rob the Cow. If only my doctor could have told me on the day I was diagnosed that a man dressed as cow would make it all a lot more doable and a lot less serious. If only we could prescribe a RtC to all cancer patients. Thanks for being the best husband.

Carless, Hannah and Emmie, my Festifeel wonder women, my dream realisers, my CAN-DOERS. Thank you for your commitment to this wild ride and for dancing under the confetti with me.

My Wholesome crew in Cornwall. You may not have seen my worst days yet, but I know you would help me get through them without hesitation.

The ocean. For letting me catch my breath again.

Kay. I wish we'd met sooner. Thank you for making me believe in myself time and time again. Thank you for listening to my doubts and fears and self-discoveries as I wrote this book. I can't wait to see what outfit you make for my twentieth Cancerversary.

Maddie. I'm so glad I listened to you about moving my care to Cornwall.

Oots, Luce and the donks, the favourite four. My therapy dogs. Thanks for dangling the many carrots (especially Canada) and dropping everything for me.

Faye. Thank you for adopting us as your friend all those years ago. You helped make change more bearable.

Sarah Brown. I know you think it's bizarre that I credit you in CoppaFeel!'s story at all, but seriously, you were one of the first people to really, REALLY believe in our mission and that will always mean so much to me and Team Boobs.

Extract Coffee Roasters, for ensuring I had enough caffeine to get this thing written and get through some late nights.

Rae, for bringing a whole new meaning to rose gardens.

The entire CoppaFeel! Family who shows up to our events, who hears our cries for help, who advocates and cheerleads and wears boob costumes and blows up balloons without questions.

All the people who have shared my story far and wide, who have helped open so many doors.

Wilhelm and Lady Marms. I didn't know that rescuing you guys essentially meant rescuing myself.

Marie Curie Hospice, Hampstead and St Joseph's Hospice, Hackney. Thank you for making me understand the true meaning of hospice care and for making me want to tell the world how brilliant and necessary hospices are.

My brain team, made up of Orla, Dr Fersht and Mr Kitchen – as well as the geniuses at Queen Square gamma knife centre. Legends, the lot of you.

Our NHS and all who work in it, I salute you, you deserve better.

Unbound is the world's first crowdfunding publisher, established in 2011.

We believe that wonderful things can happen when you clear a path for people who share a passion. That's why we've built a platform that brings together readers and authors to crowdfund books they believe in – and give fresh ideas that don't fit the traditional mould the chance they deserve.

This book is in your hands because readers made it possible. Everyone who pledged their support is listed below. Join them by visiting unbound.com and supporting a book today.

With special thanks to
Extract Coffee
  Roasters
Dr. Asha
  Umrawsingh

Supporters
Emily Abbott
Rosanne Abell
Claire Ackerman

Stephanie Adamou
Claire Adams
Mhairi Adams
Rhianna Adams
Lucy Aerts
Ameena Ahsan
  Pirbhai
Tamara Al-Jabary
Albs & the Doodle
  Donks
Laura Alderson

Jennifer Aldridge
Barbara Alexander
Jane Alexander
Yvonne Alexander
Tara Alfaddagh
Caroline Allen
Lucy Allen
Kathryn Allsopp
Ben Anderson
Rebecca Anderson
Claire Antrobus

Abigail Aris

Kari Armstrong Kennedy (Kazbah)

Sabrina Artus

Michael Ashbridge

Annie Ashwell

Catherine Astley

Henrietta Atkinson

Lynne Auton

Ellie B

Alex Bailie

Stephanie Bain

Karen Baker

Nat & Tel Baker

Rachel Baker

Ellie Baldwin

Amy Banks

Alison Banova

Guy Barker

Jodie Barker

Elisabeth Barmby

James Barnes

Nicola Barnes

Shelley Barnes

Emma Barnett

Liz Barnsdale

Carolyn Barraclough

Anna Barratt

Dia Batal

Ashleen Bateman – the strongest woman I know!

Emma Bayliss

Rach Beacham

Charlotte Beardow-Jones

Michelle Beastall

Ellie Bedford

Rozi Beecham

Sarah Beevers

Katie Bekavac

Özge Bektasoglu

Samantha Bell

Vicki Bellotte

Sarah Bence

Thea Bennun

Emma Berg

Amanda Berlyn

Laura Berry

Claire Best

Michelle Beswick

Stephanie Beverley

Sarah Bignell-Howse

Charlotte Billings

Jocelyn Bindley

Lottie Bingham

Abbie Birch

Collette Bird

Alex Birket

Julia Biro

Jessie Birtle

Rachel Bishop

Chloe Black

Tracy Black

Graham Bloomfield

Kerenza Bloomfield

Susan Blunt

Rachel Boakes

Heather Boal

Sarah Bodell

Leigh Bodman

Laurie Bolger

Alex Booth

Angela Booth

Louise Borland

Kate Boulton

Wendy Boulton

Rebecca Bowers

Hannah Bowle

Sarah Boyd

Marlene Brace

Kirsty Brade

Kim Bradford

Alice Bradshaw

Helen Brady

Kieran Brady

Holly Braine

Annie Brannan

Becky Brennan

Jess Briggs

Louisa Brinton

Stephanie Brister

Kelly Broome

Joanna Broomes

Amey Brown

Diane Brown

Jen Brown

Jodie Brown

Lorraine Brown

Clare Bryant

Poppy Buchan

Alex Buckmaster

Anna Bugg

Fleur Bugg

Hugo Bugg

Emma Bull

Paige Bull

Andrea Burden

Katrina Burge

Jessica Burke

Hannah Burn

Emma Louise
 Burnell

Emily Burton

Grace & Lily Burton

Jem Burton

Jane Bush

Susan Bushnell

Hannah Buske

MollyEllen Busker

Emma Butcher

Lizzy Butler

Molly Butler

Jill Butterwick

Jeanine Byrne

Jo Bywater

Julia Caiger-Barker

Alison Caine

Vicky Caldecourt

Nadia Calder

Lucy Caldicott

Helen Callanan

Josh Calthorpe

Alice Calvert

Hayley Campbell

Sophie Campkin

Tristan Canfer

James Cann

Vicky 'Vix' Carden
 Powell

Linda Carless

Sarah Carless

Caro

Antonia Carr

Emily Carr

Janice Carrie

Franziska Carter

Karen Carter

Rose Cashman-
 Pugsley

Caroline Cassidy

Jenna Catlin

Claire Cawte

Rebecca Channon

Jane Chapman

Christina
 Charalambous

Samantha
 Charlesworth

Zoë Charman

Kate Chartres

Rosie Checksfield

Marie Chilvers

Charlotte Chowdhry

Katie Chown

Alana Christie

Liv Christmas

Claire Clark

Gemma Clark

Vicki Clark

Thea Clausen

Beth Clayton

Jamie Clews
Annette Coates
Ruth Coglan
Laura Colbourne
Lauren Colchester
David Collier
Fiona Collier
Niamh Collins
Laura Colwell
Vicki Connerty
Helen Constantinou-
     Mantilas
Barnaby Cook
Gill Cook
Grace Cook
Hannah Cook
Laura Cook
Alice Cooke
Harry Cooke
Julie Cooke
Becky Cooper
Fiona Cooper
Trevor Coote
Han Cosham
Aya Costantino
Sayo Costantino
Anne Courso
Claire Coventry
Jenny Coventry

Kate Coventry
Jodie Cowan
Louisa Cowan
Debbie Cowling
Patrick Cox
Emily Coxhead
Verity Coyle
Katherine Crabb
Lauren Craig
Jane Craigie
Elaine Crompton
Aisling Crosland
Amanda Crowle
Joy Crowley
Victoria Cullen
Dursey Culleton
Emma Cullingford
Hanna-Liisa
     Culverwell
Emma Curtis
Frank Cussen
Nicola Cutmore
Tanya D'souza
Sarah Dale
Bjørg Dam
Sophie Danby
Rishi Dastidar
Charlotte Davies
Lian Davies

Michael Davies
Michelle Davies
Gina Davy
Alison Daw
Isabell Dawkins
Daniel Dawson
Sue De Cesare
Hayley Dean
Lou Delapena
Martinne DeMornay
Megan Denning
Rachel Derby
Susan Derbyshire
Jessica Deunert
Helen Deverell
Lisa Devine
     Tripconey
Megan Devonald
Kreena Dhiman
Caroline Dickson
Sarah Dimmock
Sarah Dixon
Hillary Dobos
Katie Dobson
Jan Doherty
Rachel Don-Leo
Sophie Dopierala
Chloe Doyle
Margaret Doyle

Nikki Doyle
Jenny Drew
David Drummond
Peter Drummond
Gemma Duff
Natalie Duffy
Chui Shuin Duke
Richard Alan Duke
Jane Duncan
Shannon Dunne
Láďa Durchánek
Sarah Earles
Naomi Eden
Simon Edhouse
Deb Edwards
Lisa Edwards
Megan Edwards
Rob Edwards
Sioned Edwards
Hannah Ellicott
Diane Ellingham
Louise Elliott
Cadell Ellis
Jeannie Ellis
Jenny and Gareth
    Ellis
Rachel Elvans
Alison Evans
Donna Evans

Lucy Evans
Sarah Evans
Natasha Faith
Squash Falconer
Elaine Fallon
Vanessa Farrell
Sara Faulkner
Caroline Feltham
Tabitha Feltham
Hannah Ferguson
Victoria Ferrer
Kate Fewkes
Zoe Field
Filiz (Filibom as my
    family call me :-))
Rachel Finch
Helen Finnis
Simon Finnis
Chloe Flain
Katherine Flannery
Jessica Fleet
Lisa Fleming
Joanna Forest
Sarah Forshaw
Dawn Foster
Julie Foster
Olivia Foster
Rebecca Foster
Leah Fountain

Sheena Fowler
Suzanne Fox
Jenna Foxton
Rachel Foye
Christopher Ear
Hats Franks
Celia Fraser
Joan Frazer
Cassandra Frey-Mills
Becky Full
Hannah Gaffey
Laura Gallagher
Edd Gamlin
Verity Gammage
Lyndsey Garrett
Lorraine Gear
Hannah Geary
Katie Geraghty
Julie Gibbon
Sarah Gibling
Emma Gibson
Nikki Gibson
Zoe Gibson Quirk
Kate Gilbert
Wendy Gillan
Anna Gillespie
Jayne Gillies
Penelope Gillings
Katy Gilmartin

Hannah-Mary
Gilroy
Faye Gishen
Carla Giudice
Lisa Givens-Rolfe
Jen Glendinning
Hollie Glover
Jayne Goddard
Susan Godfrey
Tracy Godfroy
Jennie Gollan
Abi Goswell
Lorna Goulding
Lucy Gourlay
Neil Gray
Nick Gray
Jennifer Green
Susannah Gregory
Anne Griffith
Cathy Griffiths
Lydia Griffiths
Mara Grkinic
Sarah Groezinger
Carrie Gunn
Clare Guppy
Makenna Guyler
Oa Hackett
Gemma Hall
Katrina Hallawell

Kris Hallenga
Rachel Hallett
Nicola Halsall
Alex Halstead
Gina Hamilton
Samar Hammam
Kat Hampton
Sabine Handtke
Barbara Hanna
Allie Hannah
Laura Hannon
Caz Hardiker
Jen Hardy @
mynewnormal_
Sean Harkin
Carolyn Harlow
Becca Harper-Day
Rachel Harris
Sophie Harris
Alison Paula
Harrison
Jacqueline Harrison
Megan Harrison
Lynne Harrower
Mike Harth
Ana Harvey
Elise Harvey
Em Harvey
Jo Harvey

Nat Haskell
Chelsea Haughton
Zoë Haynes
Doremi Hayward
Vaardal
Claire Hazleton
Victoria
Hebblethwaite
Richard Hedges
Angie Hegerty Ward
Sharon Henderson
Maria Henley
Jules Hennell
Helena Henshaw
Gemma Primrose
Henson
Becs Herd
Claire Heron-
Maxwell
Nicole Herridge
Jiff Heskey
Amanda Hickling
Moira Hickson
Anna Hill
Laura Hill
Rachel Hill
Natalie Hilliger
Eleanor Hindle
Nicola Hinton

Caitlin Hirst
Helen Hirst
Sarah Hodder
Sarah Hogan
Caroline Holden
Kimberley Hollas
Jennifer Hollway
Anna Holman
Emma Holt
Esme Homer
Tina Hopes
Beth Hopkins
Rhiannon Hopkins
Amy Hopwood
Kate Hosking
Lauren Howe
Eleanor Howie
Al Howman
Rebecca Hoyle
Rose Hudson
Abigail Hudspith
Marianne Huggett
Francesca Hughes
Gemma Hughes
Lea Hughes
Sarah Sunbeam
    Humphreys
Stacey Humphreys
Kathryn Humphries

Natalie Humphries
Carly Hunt
Emily Hunt
Jennifer Hunter
Stephanie Hunter
Tia-mai Hurst
Alison Hutchings
Sammy Jo Hutton
Heledd Iago
IKS
Elizabeth Ingman
Claire Inkpen
Becky Irwin
Gemma Isaac
Oliver Ivory-Bray
Kat Jackman
Estelle Jacobs
Alice Jaffray
Ailsa James
Bear James
Claire James
Rachel Jeffrey
Claudia Jenkins
Jodie Lee Jenkins
Laura Jenkins
Lorna Jenkins
Sofie Jenkinson
Jacquie Jenner
Michelle Jennings

Nelle Jervis
Debbie Jesner
Jess
Nicki John
Charlotte (Lotty)
    Johnson
Kristy Johnson
Les Johnson
Olivia Johnson
Sophie Johnson
Bethan Jones
Christine Jones
Emily Jones
Holly Jones
Michaela Jones
Phoebe Jones
Rachael Jones
Rachel Jones
Sarah J Jones
Stephen Jones
Emma Jones
    Marshall
Keely Joseph
Sophie Hannah Joy
Libby Justice
Kuda Kache
India Kahn
Eleanor Kalaher
Milan Karol

Gabrielle Kasner

Mira Kassouf

Aunty Kat-Kat

Debbie Kealey

Amy Kean

Emma Keeling

Libby Keen

Sam Keenaghan

Becca Kelly

Pauline Kelly

Kathryn Melanie
  Kemp

Louise Kempson

Christina Kennedy

Judy Kennedy

Sandra Rachel
  Kennedy

Becky Kent

Daisy Kenvin
  CoppaFeel

Aoife Kerley

Bea Kerlin

Katerina Kerouli

Dan Kieran

Katie Kierman

Emmie Kingdon

Liz Kingdon

Will Kinnaird

Linde Kirby

Lucy Kirkland

Robyn Kiy

Madeleine Koskull

Konstanze Krüger

Emma Lagarde

Elyse Lake

Abbie Lamb

Jonathan Lamb

Joanna Langton

Cole Larkin
  (Boobette)

Timur Lauer

H Lavender

Ruth Lavender

Kathy Lavis

Josie Lawrence

Nigel Lax

Dominic and
  Martha Lay

Meriel Leary

Teresa Lee

Becky Leggett

Felicity Leigh

Liz Lenagh

Jill Lethbridge

Kat Lewin-Harris

Bex Lewis

Kirsty Lewis

Laura Lewis

Lucy Lewis

Maddie Lewis

Cathy Leyland

Claudette Lilliefelth

Lisa Lindstrom

Kate Lines

Victoria Lister

Chloe Livingstone-
  Evans

Nikki Livingstone-
  Rothwell

Lorna Livock

Jonathan Lloyd

Rob Lock

Helen Lockland

Emy Loewendahl

Rach Logan

Tash Logan

Chloe Long

Abigail Longthorn

Caron Lord

Emily Lord

Lynsey Lorrance

Jemimah Loveday

Ashley Loveman

Beth Lovering

Elley Lovett

John Lowe

Krista Lowe

Amy Lucas

Kerry Luter

Debra Lyonette

Jo M

Suzanne Richmond
Maasland

Lucinda Mabbitt

Els Mac

Michelle Macartney

Chirsty Macaulay

Rachel MacBryde

Eilidh MacDonald

Holly Macdonald

Katie Macdonel

Fiona Macfarlane

Lisa Macfarlane

Alana Macfarlane
Kempner

Caitlin MacGregor

Kirsty Maclean

Iain (Tinman)
MacLeod

Annabel Maguire

Lauren Mahon

Sarah Maker

Annie Maltby

Lindsey Mander

Sarah Manning

Kathryn Mannix

Mar

Melanie Marke

Pauline Marne

Lena Marquardt

Lynn Marsden

Helen Marshall

Lucy Marshall

Rachael Marshall

Katie Mart

Jane Martin

Rachel Martin

Stace Martin

Katie Martinez Diaz

Katy Mason

Jenny Masson

Anne-Marie Materna

Kirstie Mathews

Matiya & Emily

Alice Maughan

Dean May

Sarah Emma
Mayfield

Hannah Mayling

Lucy McCahon

Nicola McCann

Alice McCartney

Claire McDonald

Hannah McDonald

Mags McDonald

Thirza McDonald

Bridget McEleney

Libby McElmeel

Shauna McGettigan

Katie McGouran

Sarah McGowan

Jean McGrogan

Tina Mcguff

Amy McGufficke

Gill McGuire

Sarah Mcloughlin

Louise McOvens

Clinton McQueen

Katy McSkimming

Jennie Mead

Sian Meades-
Williams

Hanna Meakin

Jessica Meller

Emma Melody

Emma Metcalfe

Chloe Metzger

Charlotte Meyer

Michelle

Laila Milborrow

Ivana Miletic
Demmel

Debs Millar

Amber Miller

Hannah Miller

Jo Miller

Eleanor Millsom

Joanna Mitchell

John Mitchinson

Graham Moates

Franny Mobbs

Lynne Mollison

Alastair Monk

Kerri Monk

Lizzie Monk

Claire Montgomery

Michelle Mooney

  – for Joanne

Heather Moore

Jodi Morgan

Elan Morris

Gemma Morris

Hannah Morris

Melissa Morris

Rachel Morris

Rachel Moss

Natalie Mounsey

Becky Mount

Rachel Mowat

Miranda Mowbray

Marian Moylan

Gail Muller

Danielle Munday

Isobel Munro

Bree Murdock

Hannah Murray

Jasmin Myhill

Rebecca Naisby

Lynn Napier

Julie Narramore

Natasha Nash

Brenda Nasr

Carlo Navato

Poppy Naylor

Amy Neill

Sophia Neuhaus

Emma Newman

Verena Newton

Helen Nicell

Karen Nicholl

Hazel Nicholson

Kerry Nicholson

Tess Nicholson

Nicola

Erinn Nicolson

Danielle Niepold

Mike Niles

Shirley Nolan

Amee Norman

Karen Norris

Amanda Norrlander

Jenni North

Pat Noto

Lisa O'Connell

Tim O'Connor

Sarah O'Neill

Robyn O'Brien

Charlotte O'Connor

Carrie O'Donnell

Poppy O'Rourke-

  Burr

Philippa Ogle

Kate OHara

Becky Okell

Judy Osman

Rosie Osmaston

Saskia Osterloff

Tracy Ostridge

Denise OSullivan

Joelle Owusu-

  Sekyere

Dominique Paduch

Alicia Page

Danni Page

Emma Palmer

Amy Parker

Ellie Parker

Rebecca Parker

Rachel Parks

Victoria Parnell Reid

Craig Parsons

Olga Paskins

Olivia Pass

Jess Patching

Bianca Paterson

Michaela Peacock

Laura Pearce

Emer Pearson

Louise Pearson

Millie Pearson

Nicola Peck

Victoria Penko

Hayley Pennington

Beth Penny

Louis Perry

Noo Pert

Lilli Peters

Victoria Pettitt

Naomi Phillips

Rhiannon Phillips

Kay Phoenix

Olivia Pickerill

Ellen Pickett

Kelly Pietrangeli

Alice Pike

Zanna Pill

Nancy Pilon

Tracey Pinfold

Elsie Pinniger

Gemma Pitchford

Christine Podesta

Justin Pollard

Ildiko Polyak

Louise Pontefract

Katherine Poole

Kirsty Poole

Marianna Popejoy

Mary Porter

Amber Postings

Anna Potamianou

Kerry Potter

Megan Potts

Alice Powell

Sandy Powell

Jo Powis

Michèle Poynter

Isabel Preston

Laura Price

Nicola Price

Sarah Prinold

Ruth Prior

Ginny Purcell

Alice-May Purkiss

Emma Pyper

Patricia Qadir

Judith Quinn

Tracy Raine

Holly Rawlings

Claire Ray

Kate Ray

Freya Ray Brown

Alex Recio

Millie Rees

Samantha Reeve

Charlotte Reeves

Emma Reynolds

Natalie Reynolds

Lizzie Rhymes

Beth Richard

Kate Rickett

Anna Riley

Jessica Riley

Zoe Rippingale

Hollie Robbins

Ellie Robins

Beth Robinson

Emily Robson

Jennie Roddy

Laura Roe

Laura Rolls

Lyddie Rose

Anna Ross

Eleanor Ross

Eve Rossi

Jess Rourke

Aimee Rowe-Best

Becky Rowell

Hayley Rowland

Millie Ruck

Tom Ruddell

Charlotte Rush

Claire Russell

Holly Rutherford

Lisa Ryan

Sarah Salisbury

Ashleigh Salter

Christoph Sander

John Sanders

Chloe Sandiford

Lesley Sands

Eve Saunders

Emma Scott

Joan Scott

Jackie Scully

Emily Seaborn

Madi Seabrook

Anne Sebert

Arthur Sebert

Kay Sennitt

Leah Sharpe

Bryony Shaw

Emma Shaw

David Shelley

Anna Shepherd

Clare Sherman

Josh Shinner

Jenny Shipley

Laura Shorc

Lauren Shortland

Samantha Shrubb

Jackie Silva

Felicity Sirc

Elaine Slater

Nicola Slawson

Ngadi Smart

Andrew Smith

Caroline Smith

Cliff Smith

Emma Smith

Euan Smith

Hanna Smith

Holly Smith

Karen Smith

Liberty Smith

Liz Smith

Sandra Smith

Steffi Smith

Valarie Smith

Lou Smith MA

Krystyna Smolinski

Alice Solomoms

Sarah Somerset

Leanne Southern

Chelsea Sowden

Helen Spencer

Avie Stalker

Zoe Stamp

Kayleigh Stapleton

Amanda Steele

Tracie Steeley

Katie Steingold

Catherine Stephen

Jessica Stephens

Emily Stevens

Fiona Stewart

Jo Stewart

Melissa Stiles

Hazel Stinson

Chloe Stockley

Bel Stone

Elli Stone

Lauren Stone

Lynn Stonehouse

Beth Stoneman

Francesca Storti

Stephen Stretton

Tara Stubington

Beth-Louise Sturdee

Pippa Suren

Jennifer Sutcliffe

Jessica Sutherland

Laurie-ann
    Sutherland

Dawn Svenson
    Holland

Angela Swain
Belinda Swan
Laura Swandel
Amy Swanson
Michelle Sykes
Bronagh Synnott
Emily Talling
Tia Tamblyn
Laura Tannahill
Tapi Kudz Taruvinga
Claire Taylor
Juliette Taylor
Kim Taylor
Lisa Taylor
Lizzie Taylor
Lucy Taylor
Annabelle Teale
Kimberley Teale
Keeley Tempest
Lauren Terry
Felicity Theaker
Hannah Theaker
Carly Theodosi
Anna Thomas
Victoria Thomas
Lucy Thompson
Samantha Thompson
Sarah Thompson
Sinéad Thompson

Fiona Thomson
Jessica Thomson
Lucy Thorman
Abbi Thorpe
Ruth Till
Lauren Timperley
Shelley Titmus
Alan David Tollan
Katie Tombs
Amber Tomkins
Hannah Tomkins
Susan Tomlin
Emily Tonkin
Nicole Tootill
Pippa Torbett
Dina Torkia
Zoe Towers
Jen Townsend
Katherine Tracey
Soph Trew
Katerina Tsang
Diana Tsyporyna
Matthew Tubbs
Becky Turland
Faye Turner
Gemma Turner
Hana Turšič
Beth Upton
Cara Upton

Aisling Vaughan
Loubie Vaughan
Elaine Vece
Bojana Vilus
Emily Vinnicombe
Chrissy Voigt
Laura Waddilove
Emily Wakeland
Claire Walbrin
Leanne Waldron
Eilidh Walker
Jennifer Walker
Megan Walker
Ciara Wall
Laura Walsh
Claire Wanless
Emma Ward
Gemma Ward
Lydia Ward
Lorna Ward-Webster
Debbie Warner
Lucy Warwood
Cassie Waters
Carolyn Waterworth
Laura Watkins
Zeta Watkins
Annabel Watson
Eleanor Watson
Kirsty Watson

Mhairi Watson

Lucy Watts

Carolyn Webb

Rachel Webb

Sharmaine Webley

Zoë Webster

Maire Welham

Lauren Wellby

Vicki Weston

Jessie Whalley

Carolyn Whincup

Olivia Whinton

Rhiannon Whitby

Elise White

Kate White

Katharine White

Isabel Whitehead

Abigail Whitehouse

Beverley Whitlock

Trevor Whittaker

Victoria Whittaker

Nicola Wiggins

Chaniece Wild

Natasha Wilkinson

Christen Williams

Emma Williams

Emma Ceris
  Williams

Laura Williams

Lauren Williams

Charlotte Williamson

Jo Williamson

Danielle Willis

Anna Wilson

Claie Wilson

Katherine Wilson

Liz Wilson

Sal Wilson

Lady Wilson
  McBoob Of
  Titville and Nork
  Twin Faces

Helen Wingate

Dorothy Wingrove

Ellie Winter

Emma Winter

The Wolfwoods

Fearne Wood

Kirsty Wood

Robyn Wood

Alex Woodfield

Bexy Woodside

Julie Worrall

Jo Wright

Sara Wright

Debbie Wythe

Suzi Yazdi

Steve Shad Yelland

Maho Yokoyama

Michelle Young

Yvie Young

PierGiorgio Zucco

Susan Zwinkels

Heidi Zymela